What Your Doctor Won't
(or Can't) Tell You

What Your Doctor Won't (or Can't) Tell You

DOCTORS, HOSPITALS, DRUGS,
INSURANCE — WHAT YOU NEED TO
KNOW TO TAKE CHARGE OF
YOUR OWN HEALTH CARE

Evan Scott Levine, MD

G. P. PUTNAM'S SONS
NEW YORK

⫿P

G. P. Putnam's Sons
Publishers Since 1838
a member of
Penguin Group (USA) Inc.
375 Hudson Street
New York, NY 10014

Library of Congress Cataloging-in-Publication Data

Levine, Evan Scott.
What your doctor won't (or can't) tell you : doctors, hospitals, drugs, insurance—what you need to know to take charge of your own health / Evan Scott Levine
p. cm.
Includes bibliographical references.
ISBN 0-399-15150-8
1. Levine, Evan Scott.   2. Medical care—Miscellanea.
3. Medical errors.   4. Cardiologists—Biography.   I. Title.
RA395.A3L485   2004   2003058576
362.1'0973—dc22

Printed in the United States of America
1   3   5   7   9   10   8   6   4   2

This book is printed on acid-free paper. ∞

Book design by Chris Welch

*This book is dedicated to my patients
and to those of you whose greatest enjoyment in life
is helping a fellow human being or an animal
in need—in spite of any risks.*

Contents

What Your Doctor Won't
(or Can't) Tell You

Introduction

I have been a practicing cardiologist and internist in the state of New York for the last twelve years.

I enjoy a sterling reputation, and I take great pride in my work. Yet, for some time now I have been growing increasingly discontented and, more to the point, disturbed about the direction and the deterioration of modern medicine in this country. When I turned forty last year, I decided the time had come to do something I had only talked about with friends and colleagues for the last decade. I decided to write an informative, utterly truthful, and no-holds-barred book about what has happened to the practice of medicine in the United States of America, no matter what the consequences might be for me. I want to tell you what you can do, as a medical consumer, to get the very best treatment when you are suddenly taken ill or are diagnosed with a serious, life-threatening illness or are seeking a second opinion or are in search of a new primary-care physician, or have a loved one who is facing one of these problems.

I am an insider. Like many troubled insiders in other professions, I could just keep my mouth shut and look the other way. But it is high time someone blew the whistle. I want to tell you what you may have suspected, or what you have surely read about in bits and pieces, for years. We doctors have been silent for too long. Too many of us in the field of medicine are scared. Scared to rock the boat, scared of retribution, scared of doing damage to our livelihoods. Others, too many others, are more interested in getting rich than they are in helping their patients get well.

I do not intend in these pages to stitch together just the cautionary tales and scary stories you might read about in the newspaper or see on television, but rather to convey the real story of the largest and most complex profession, science, and business in this country. Medicine, you see, is no longer best portrayed by one of those charming posters by Norman Rockwell you might still see in your doctor's or your child's pediatrician's office. On the contrary—as most of you must know from your less than satisfactory encounters within the system—the medical *industry* has become a monolithic moneymaking machine. What began long ago as a simple relationship between a doctor and his patient has turned into a commercialized, profoundly cynical, and intrinsically perverse (I am tempted to say *unwell*) profession that is gobbling up billions of dollars of our nation's wealth and distributing an unfair share of it to the huge insurance and pharmaceutical corporations, conglomerated hospital corporations (for profit *and* not for profit), money-grubbing physicians, and duplicitous lawyers.

As I write these words, there are things about the medical profession that sadden and frighten me, even upset me to the point where I have trouble getting a good night's sleep. There are people in the business of medicine who are causing our insurance premiums to skyrocket, denying us the decent health care we deserve, and cheating our government. Many of them have become very rich, and in so doing they have bastardized the originating ideology of my profession and the sacred oath of Maimonides, which reads:

> The eternal providence has appointed me to watch over the life and health of Thy creatures. May the love for my art actuate me at all time; may neither avarice nor miserliness, nor thirst for glory or for a great reputation engage my mind; for the enemies of truth and philanthropy could easily deceive me and make me forgetful of my lofty aim of doing good to Thy children.
>
> May I never see in the patient anything but a fellow creature in pain.
>
> Grant me the strength, time and opportunity always to correct what I have acquired, always to extend its domain; for knowledge is immense and the spirit of man can extend indefinitely to enrich itself daily with new requirements.
>
> Today he can discover his errors of yesterday and tomorrow he can obtain a new light on what he thinks himself sure of today. Oh, God, Thou has appointed me to watch over the life and death of Thy creatures; here am I ready for my vocation and now I turn unto my calling.

There are competing special-interest groups that seek to divert appropriate funds from research into one disease to another. For example, diabetes and heart disease kill far more women every year than breast cancer, yet few medical professionals or politicians are brave enough to confront this.

I receive letters and calls from shameless entrepreneurs—many of whom have entered the newly burgeoning imaging market—promising me hundreds of dollars for each patient I send to their office. Others—unaffiliated with the manufacturer of Botox—call to ask if I wish to earn extra money by giving Botox injections to patients. While many say no to such unethical procedures, too many others say yes. I know of many physicians who are performing, or at least billing for, studies that they have never been trained to do and should not be doing. And these above-mentioned imaging businesses (many owned by physicians) now tell you they can scan your entire body with their newfangled machines in the local mall and find cancer or heart disease before it causes you any trouble. Yet they don't mention that many of these studies will prove to be incorrect and send you and your family down a lengthy and tortuous path of additional expense, fear, and dread, not to mention more and more tests. Even the very well-respected Society of Thoracic Radiology issued a consensus statement on screening for lung cancer by this technique (often referred to as low-dose helical CT). It recommends against such procedures until and unless benefits to patients are validated by appropriate trials.[1] Centers like these are not approved by any qualified supervisory society, and yet they are open for business to take your and/or your insurer's money.

I know of unqualified physicians who are performing imaging studies, angiography, and even surgery in order to fill their pockets with money. They can rationalize this conflict of interest quite well today. The procedure might be entirely paid by a patient's insurance company, and what's more, perhaps the person even asked for it. After all, doctors don't want to miss anything or to be accused of a misdiagnosis, or else the malpractice attorney will be on them like a vulture on carrion. The majority of my experience is in the field of cardiology, but in my opinion over half of all imaging studies in our country are performed without meeting clearly defined published guidelines. Some are done because the physician is a dolt, others to prevent a potential lawsuit, but the great majority occur because the doctor has just found an easy way to make more money.

There are many gifted physicians who also perform other unnecessary studies. Cardiac catheterizations are an epidemic in this country, as are arthroscopic surgeries. In the July 2002 *New England Journal of Medicine,* a randomized single-blind study concluded that arthroscopic surgery performed on patients with degenerative arthritis is useless.[2] Yet several hundred thousand of these procedures at well over $1,000 apiece are performed every year. Both my mom and dad had this surgery.

Doctors are also making illicit deals with other doctors, and in extraordinary numbers. Too many are out for themselves or, at the very least, have been made cynical and uncaring by the system in which they are mired. But not all of them. Indeed, there are still many brilliant and caring physicians yearning to make people healthy and happy. You just have to know how and where to find them, and that is the other main thrust of this book.

When I entered a medical school program at age eighteen in 1979, physicians were still considered pillars of the community and, with a few rare exceptions, above reproach. Medicine was a noble calling, and I was proud to be entering such a tradition. I grew up in a middle-class neighborhood in the borough of Brooklyn, in New York City. My hard-working, blue-collar parents scrimped and saved to give me everything I needed and encouraged me to study and reap the rewards that a good education could bring.

I received my medical degree and graduated summa cum laude after completing a six-year program affiliated with the City College of New York and Mount Sinai School of Medicine. I then interned and completed my residency in medicine as well as cardiology at Montefiore Medical Center in the Bronx, New York. Currently, I have offices in the Bronx and in Yonkers, New York, and I am affiliated with Montefiore Medical Center, where I am a clinical assistant professor of medicine. I also have an assistant professorship at the Tauro School for Physician Assistants. I am board certified in both internal medicine and cardiology, and I have admitting privileges at two community hospitals in Yonkers.

Reward was and thankfully still remains my great satisfaction when I help someone—a stranger, a friend, or sometimes even a family member—get better. Yet what the public is not aware of is that often the worst sort of physicians, members of what I can only call a criminal element that has infiltrated this once great profession, are reaping the largest of the monetary rewards. No study can tell you this, but it is the talk among the good, honest physicians today, and unfortunately it is the truth.

Equally pathetic are the pariahs—the lawyers—who hope to win the lottery for themselves and their clients at the expense of the physician (even though often no malpractice has been committed) and the public. These awards continue to drive up the cost of malpractice insurance to all physicians, while they also create a great amount of fear and mistrust in what was once a sacred doctor/patient relationship. We all have a finite life span and all medical procedures have known complications, yet the most unscrupulous lawyers can turn any case into a million-dollar settlement.

I've decided that I can no longer stand by and watch all this happen. And as much as I intend to be a whistleblower in these pages, I also want to give the best possible guidance about how people can make their way successfully through the medical system as a patient. In Chapter 1, "How to Choose Your Doctor," I urge you to seek out only the best physicians and suggest proven ways for you to find them. You should avoid the crafty charlatan who may have the largest advertisement in the local Yellow Pages or the most pressing ad campaign. The days of choosing a doctor and leaving it up to him are over, and yet many of us still do more research regarding the purchase of a new car or appliance than we do when it comes to our own health-care providers and our illnesses. But all doctors are not created equal. Some physicians are much more intelligent than others, some are more caring, some more greedy and duplicitous. It is my fervent hope that the stories I tell will provoke people into devoting more time and energy to this crucial and, in some cases, life-or-death process of choosing a physician, and that if you find you are not satisfied with your doctor after reading these pages, you will get a new one.

In Chapter 2, "How to Survive Your Hospital Stay," you will read about the dangers all patients face when they are hospitalized. You'll be informed about ways of finding a good-quality hospital and, once you are there, obtaining the care that will make you better instead of sicker. Hospitals are facing difficult times right now, and many have made a decision, probably for financial reasons, to cut back on the quality of care. Since hospitals are now paid by the insurance companies based on a patient's diagnosis (called a DRG code), regardless of the length of his or her stay, most hospitals have recruited specially trained workers whose sole job it is to coax the doctor into discharging the patient as soon as possible—sometimes sooner than is safe or advisable—in order to free the bed for the next paying patient. Hospitals now actually publish lists (their equivalent of a Hall of Shame, I guess) meant to embarrass the physicians whose average patient's length of stay is considered too long and have administrators call their offices asking them to discharge their patients at the first possible opportunity. Some physicians, so intimidated by these calls and published lists, are persuaded to send a patient home a bit too early or to a nursing home for continued, albeit lower-quality, care. I have endured instances where, had I not been unyielding and, frankly, even bellicose in reaction to such pressures from above, my patient might well have died as a result.

Hospital food, as we all know, has become atrocious, worse than what prisoners are served in jail. Nurses have been replaced by technicians in white uniforms, and many highly qualified physicians have been replaced by those who will or must accept a lower salary. Most hospital administrators meet with their doctors regularly, not to discuss how to improve health care but rather how to encourage the physician to see more patients in less time. What makes all of this truly appalling is that these facts contrast so glaringly with the barrage of recent commercials that hospitals broadcast depicting their centers as places of caring.

Hard as it may be to believe, some hospitals, including Columbia Presbyterian in New York City, now actually require all voluntary physicians to sign a contract giving the hospital 10 percent of their income if they wish to admit their patients there.[3] Recently, Dr. Gerald Fischbach, dean of the faculty of medicine at Columbia, was quoted in the *New York Times*[4] about this mandatory tax/extortion. "'There is a tax, if you want to call it a tax,'" said Dr. Fischbach of the $12.5 million in funds that he controls. "'I call it a contribution. It is a tax levied on physicians on their income to help the place run.'" Smaller hospitals sometimes take the opposite tack and actually bribe physicians to stay and admit their patients to their hospitals. They give these physicians salaried positions that compensate the doctors beyond the amount of work they perform for the hospital.

The pharmaceutical industry has discovered many important drugs that have saved the lives of countless millions of people, but they have also been rewarded with handsome profits from the sale of these drugs. In Chapter 6, "The Pharmaceutical Industry," you will learn how these same companies have manipulated the price and utilization of their products in the prescription-drug market, and how they send their representatives into doctors' offices and hospitals to pressure physicians into using their drugs instead of those of their competitors. Physicians are being pressured every day to use brand-name prescription drugs (which may be ten times the cost and possibly not as efficacious as generic prescription drugs) by reps who are paid their salaries based upon the number of prescriptions written for their drug in their territory. Incentives are so significant that these sales-people might earn more money than the physicians they call on if they sell their product well.

It is clear to me that a complete overhaul of the pharmaceutical industry is in order. At the very least, the entire field-rep system, where wheedling, cajoling, and, yes, special incentives are common, must be eliminated. In return, what are often absurd class-action suits against a particular drug that reward billions of dollars to lawyers and patients must be stopped. These handouts—often in complete violation of the scientific data—cost all of us more when it comes to the medications that we need to have.

Besides being an exposé of the industry, the information provided in Chapter 6 should help you obtain the best medication at the most reasonable price. You'll be given examples of medications that are equally as efficacious in treating an ailment yet far from equal in the price you pay for them.

I have also included a chapter on the tricks of the trade or how some unscrupulous doctors sell you services, drugs, and even operations that you don't need. In another chapter, you will read about why I strongly advise you always to get a second opinion. I'll also explain why you should always avoid the temptation of taking part in a clinical study unless there is the most obvious and significant benefit to you and not only to the investigator, who is often paid up to $5,000 by a pharmaceutical company for studying the effects of that drug on you. I conclude with a chapter on medicine in a state of crisis, about what it is like to be a doctor in these most trying times for our profession.

I hope you and the members of your family will read this book carefully and use it as a guide and as an inspiration to help you get the best possible medical care, whether the need arises as the result of an auto accident, a life-threatening illness, a routine checkup, or a second opinion. Perhaps if we all understood more about the risks and pitfalls inherent in the system as it exists today, and the benefit or lack of benefit of expensive tests, not to mention the importance of preventive medicine, we could dramatically improve the quality of health care in this country and lower its skyrocketing costs. I hope that this book provides an impetus to some of us to do just that.

I want to wake up America and revolutionize the health-care system. Hospitals should be required to provide patients with clean, quiet rooms and three quality meals a day. Physicians, not administrators, need to make decisions about the withholding of care or the discharge of a patient. Hospitals need to be policed more carefully by outside government agencies with the authority to make changes.

In addition, malpractice suits should fit the name—*malpractice*—not *poor outcome*. We need to realize that malpractice attorneys have infiltrated the health-care system through advertisements of huge settlements and the 1-800 commercialization of a once-honorable profession. These lawyers are out to collect a third of any settlement through any means and at a great cost to our health-care system. Their manipulation of the public, the media, and nonprofessional jurors has tainted the patient/

physician relationship and markedly increased the cost of your health care. Good physicians as well as bad ones are being sued in record numbers. Any lawsuit, whether won or lost, is very costly to a physician, who must sit in a courtroom, sometimes for weeks, while his practice and patients are ignored. A professional panel should be given the charge of deciding what penalty (financial or criminal) should be weighed against the physician, and reasonable financial awards should be set.

I dedicate this book to all of those who have suffered at the hands of our health-care system, both patients and physicians, and I thank the many individuals I have known who have inspired me to be myself and be the best health-care provider I can possibly be.

CHAPTER 1

How to Choose Your Doctor

How do you choose your doctor? It's not a very easy question to answer. However, I can tell you how *not* to choose your physician and, if nothing else, give you a tried-and-true set of guidelines as you make one of the most important decisions of your life.

I have been told many times by my patients and even my friends that when they are suddenly in need of medical attention or advice they simply open up the Yellow Pages and pick the physician with the largest advertisement. Needless to say, this is not a good way to find an excellent doctor. Or a plumber, for that matter. Others have told me that they close their eyes and pick their physician from the pages of their HMO book. Think about that for a moment: putting your life into the hands of a stranger picked at random out of the Yellow Pages or from some health-care provider's booklet. Would you buy a car or appliance using this method? When you purchase a car, don't you go automatically to *Consumer Reports* to check out the reviews and ratings and then give it a test drive first? One of the most important things you can do after reading this chapter if you do not yet have a primary doctor is to go find one before you get ill. Looking for a physician when you are sick with a fever or, God forbid, a much more serious ailment is not an opportune time to start.

The first thing to consider is the qualifications of the primary-care physician or specialist. Although medical credentials do not always guarantee a physician's knowledge and expertise, they are a good place to start. So find out where the doctor went to medical school and where he or she did his or her residency. This information can be obtained by looking in books like *Who's Who in Medicine and Health Care,* by calling your local hospital, or simply by calling the doctor's office.[1] You can also use the *U.S. News & World Report* website (*www.usnews.com*), for example, to find out a great deal more about medical-school rankings. I know my staff is always eager to answer these questions. Yet when I called a handful of offices in the five boroughs of New York City, I found that some of them were reluctant to answer my questions. In such instances, one can only surmise that these offices were staffed by physicians with second-rate training and dubious skills. Again, good-quality physicians with quality staff should be not only able to answer these questions but happy to do so.

Call a few offices, especially in large medical centers, and see if you get a headache listening to the phone ringing endlessly without an answer. If you can't get through to an office to set up an appointment or to ask a simple question, imagine how you will feel when you really need to speak to the doctor. I'm sure there are patients and doctors reading this who have experienced this: no answer or an abrupt forward into a byzantine voice-mail system (often the black hole).

If you end up in an emergency room with a real medical problem, you may be given the doctor on call. The physician to whom you are assigned might be a poor doctor, indeed. The nurses in the ER are almost certainly aware of his deficiencies and are sympathetic to your dilemma, but no doubt they would be unwilling or afraid to tell you. I cannot stress enough the importance, if at all possible, of going to an ER in a large teaching hospital. You will be assigned a medical resident, and after seeing him, if you are able, you can ask him to call a physician he trusts.

While we are on the subject, perhaps the best people to ask about which doctors are super and which ones are not are the medical residents and the nursing staff in an academic or teaching hospital. They know which physicians are bright and caring. They see which physician comes to see the patient in a timely manner and orders appropriate tests and consults. Or which stops by on the weekend to see what's up. But there is still that terrible code of silence I mentioned previously. It exists in all the hospitals where I have worked and studied. The staff knows which physicians to avoid yet they cannot advise the patient or his family. They could, however, if asked, suggest a physician whom you could see once you come to the hospital. Or perhaps you could prevail upon one of the nurses for her recommendation as to which physician she would see if she were in your shoes.

Being an absolute iconoclast and a true patient advocate, I have in many circumstances, and behind closed doors, told patients seeing particular specialists to get a second opinion. Or, in other words, I've told them to seek care with a doctor better qualified than the one they were seeing.

As incredible as this will sound, you also must make sure that the physician is board certified. Board certification means simply that your physician has passed a standardized test given by the nationally recognized specialty board. Frankly, in my opinion, physicians who cannot pass their board exam should not be allowed to practice their specialty. The exam is quite easy, and only 20 percent of doctors fail on their first attempt to pass it. And yet I know physicians who specialize in cardiology and pulmonary medicine, for example, who have failed their board exams several times before finally passing or who have never passed the exam at all. Statistics like these are not available, unfortunately, as I can imagine there are few potential patients who would happily submit to care by one of these frequent failures. Perhaps the simplest way to determine if your physician is board certified is to go to the site *www.abms.org*. There is no cost to register, and you can look up as many as five physicians per day.

In general, a physician must renew his certification every ten years, although many older physicians do not, probably due to some sort of grandfather clause that gives them special dispensation.

If the doctor is not board certified, then obviously I recommend that you go elsewhere, since this usually means the physician in question lacks the aptitude to pass an exam. Once again, just because the physician specializes in a particular field does not mean he is board certified.

If you walk into a physician's office and you notice that it is dirty or shabbily furnished or poorly lit or that the staff is not courteous, attentive, and professional, then I would suggest you turn right around and leave. Use your instincts, as you would in any number of situations. If you meet the physician and he looks in any way less than presentable, or seems overworked or distracted, or doesn't seem to be listening to you when you are talking to him, then I would not go back. You would be surprised, for example, to know how many MDs can be found daytrading stocks in the back office while not seeing patients. Meeting people and forming opinions about their integrity and competence is a crucial skill for us all, needless to say.

I would also take a look at the doctor's stethoscope. This is the tool of his trade. A top-of-the-line stethoscope costs less than $200. So if you see a stethoscope with pink tubing or perhaps a drug logo on it (usually a $5 stethoscope given to the physician by a pharmaceutical rep), I would be very wary. In fact, if you don't know what kind of stethoscope your doctor is using, ask him. I'm troubled by the number of physicians, even cardiologists, who use cheap and inferior stethoscopes in order to save a hundred bucks. Can you imagine such a thing? But a seemingly insignificant detail like this might save you from going to the wrong physician.

I recently came across a neurologist who did not have a bloodpressure cuff in his office. He called me to tell me that my patient was complaining of a headache during his exam. When I asked him to take her blood pressure, he replied, "I don't have a BP machine in my office." Any physician you see should be able to take your blood pressure, and most should take it as part of their exam. If you see a physician who cannot take your blood pressure I would question whether he is truly capable of taking care of his patients—or you.

Lots of us hear about doctors from our friends, but I would not rely on a friend's recommendation of a physician unless he has done his homework and you trust him implicitly. Just because someone you know has been using the same doctor for a decade does not mean that he or she is getting good care. People see doctors for twenty years and have good relationships with them but may be receiving the worst sort of care. Perhaps the only exception to this rule would be a recommendation of a good plastic surgeon, since you can at least judge with your own eyes the results of his or her work.

If you need to be referred to a specialist, all of the previous suggestions still apply. Unless it is an emergency, however, I would suggest that you ask your primary-care physician to give you the names of two physicians he would consider sending you to and then ask him if he would recommend one over the other, and if so, why. I am no longer shocked when I ask a patient why his doctor sent him to me and he tells me that he has no idea. There is an uncanny degree of blind faith at work here. Over and over again, I see the same tacit assumption made by patients of both sexes, of all ages, of all levels of education, and from all walks of life, namely that every individual with a physician's shingle hanging out in front of his or her office is equally talented, insightful, and trustworthy. Do you make the same assumption about lawyers? Or accountants? Even your electrician?

When you do choose a doctor you should also consider who your doctor works with or who covers him (takes calls in his absence) when he is not working. Since it's impossible for your doctor to work every single night and weekend, most physicians arrange what is called cross-coverage. In other words, competing doctors agree to work and cover their competitor's patients and vice versa. Sadly, there are instances (rare, one can only hope) when a bright, hardworking physician might be involved in a coverage agreement with one who is inept and unqualified. In one hospital where I attend, for example, specialists who are board certified are sometimes covered by some less-than-astute physicians who have never passed their board exams. My partners and I were involved for a very short while with another cardiologist who approached us for a coverage arrangement. One night when he was covering for us, he refused to go to the hospital to take care of a very sick patient who was having a life-threatening heart attack. At 2:00 A.M. I was tracked down by the patient's internist, who told me that the physician covering refused to go see the patient. I went in myself and took care of him. The next day, of course, we told that physician we would no longer be involved in a cross-coverage arrangement with him. As I understand it, this character is no longer practicing medicine in the United States.

So remember, when you do choose a doctor of any kind, ask him if he is involved in some sort of coverage arrangement with other physicians. Ask him for the names of those doctors and then find out if they are board certified. You might also ask your doctor if you could call him in special circumstances when his associate's coverage is not helpful. Or, to avoid this cross-coverage issue altogether, you could find a doctor you trust and respect who works in a larger group of affiliated physicians and then become familiar with all the doctors in that practice.

If you are also a patient of a specialist, like a cardiologist, your other choice if your primary-care physician is away or unavailable, or if the cross-coverage falls through or is unsatisfactory, would be to call the specialist who knows you. Many patients call me when their family doctor is not available.

There are times when your doctor, dentist, or podiatrist might sell his practice. In fact, it is illegal for a physician to "sell" his patients, and in any event, the buyer understands that the patients can always decide to leave him when the deal is made or at any time thereafter. Sometimes, however, the physician who is leaving is paid a percentage of the monies the new doctor collects over the next year. With this financial incentive in mind, the retiring doctor has a great incentive to keep you from leaving the practice. So if your doctor decides to leave or retire or to sell his practice, don't stay if you think the new doctor is not the right one for you. In fact, I would evaluate him or her just as I have suggested you evaluate every new physician. If you decide to leave, remember to get your old records, or at least a copy of them, no matter what the charge may be. (I believe it can be no more than 75¢ per copy, but most offices will charge you far less.)

There are any number of common situations I would urge you to avoid. Doctors with different areas of expertise who share offices often (but not always) have some sort of incentive to send patients to their colleague down the hall. So, unless you trust your doctor implicitly, I would avoid these situations. Frankly, in the interests of complete disclosure, one of my partners happens to be a gastroenterologist. But in order to avoid even the slightest possible appearance of bias, I tell my patients that he is a partner of mine and, if they wish, I will be more than happy to send them to another highly qualified and respected stomach doctor. In order not to influence them in any way, I do not even tell them that I send members of my own family to see him.

Husband-and-wife teams present essentially the same problem. And if your primary-care doctor tells you that a number of different specialists rent space one day a week in his offices, I would caution you that this often means some sort of shenanigans are going on.

Never call an 800 number advertised by your hospital. These advertisements remind me of the ones politicians put forth every election year, full of half-truths at best. Hospitals do this to get their physicians, most of whom are on salary at the hospital, more patients, by which I mean *more business*. I would be especially careful of small community hospitals that advertise in this way. The hospital may purchase time on a local station and make all sorts of dubious claims: We have a heart center, or wound center, or perhaps a special sleep or cancer center. Yet there is no special certificate or prestigious award to back up their claim that their center is one of excellence. Once the listener calls in, an operator gives him or her the number of a physician affiliated with that hospital. Often these doctors are picked at random from a list and again only because the hospital hopes to profit from them. I am embarrassed and outraged by these sorts of lies and distortions I hear every day on the radio as I drive to work.

The truth is that almost every hospital advertises, and even the more prestigious ones are not opposed to painting a picture of excellence even when that may be far from the case. Very often this advertising centers on the formation of a new heart or cancer center, for example, or draws attention to the arrival of a much sought after and very highly paid new physician who, the ads suggest, virtually walks on water.

On December 15, 2002, the *New York Post* ran an article titled "Hospital Heartache" that illustrates precisely the point I am trying to make. The author begins by describing how aggressively Mount Sinai Hospital marketed their new "world-renowned team" of top cardiothoracic surgeons.

"The best just got better," the ad boomed in large type.

After reading the *Post* article, however, you might conclude that Mount Sinai would rather not have had to endure this latest round of free publicity, for it went on to state that "the state Health Department is investigating complications in 28 heart procedures, including bypass surgeries and valve replacements, at the hospital earlier this year (2002)—including 21 deaths." According to the *Post*, one of the cases under investigation involved Mount Sinai's new chief of cardiothoracic surgery, Dr. David Adams, and whether he incorrectly had placed a prosthetic heart valve in a patient, who died shortly after.[2]

In November 2002, in a letter obtained by the *Post*, "the State asked Mount Sinai President Larry Hollier to explain the hospital's 'unusually high' 6.12 percent mortality rate for bypass surgery in the first half of this year." Pointing out that this mortality rate (while not adjusted for risk factors) was "substantially higher than the statewide average" (2.24 percent in 1999), the state also asked the hospital to take "corrective action."

When the *Post* reporter asked the hospital about these results, they replied that their surgical outcomes were getting better and mentioned that out "of 130 bypass operations since July, no patients have died." But Mount Sinai didn't mention that 130 by-pass cases is an unusually small number of cases to have occurred in such a large medical center during that period of time. So while I'm not sure how they lowered their surgical mortality, they might have turned away the high-risk cases instead of doing a better job.

" 'They're still a great team,' " Gary Rosenberg, executive vice president of Mount Sinai Medical Center, said of the heart surgeons, adding that "it takes a while" for a new group to get established.[3]

This investigation has not been concluded as of my writing, but Mr. Rosenberg's statement says volumes about the arrogance of such an institution.

When a hospital or medical center recruits a highly paid doctor to join its staff, that institution very quickly has to justify the large cash outlay it has made. Therefore other members of the faculty are encouraged, and in some cases pressured, to send patients to him, even though those doctors may not know if he's a good doctor or not. Recently, a very highly paid doctor, José P. García, and his team were recruited to run a new heart transplant program at Montefiore Medical Center in New York City. With millions of hospital dollars invested in this new program, it won't surprise you to learn that the hospital did not publicize the doctor's surgical mortality rate when he practiced in another state.[4] (You can rest assured that if it had been low, it would have been *publicized*.) You might assume, though, if you were a trusting sort of person and given all the hoopla, that his mortality rate was stupendously low. But here's the thing: For the year

2000, the doctor's in-house mortality rate, as reported by the Pennsylvania Health Care Cost Containment Council, was 10.3 percent, when the average or expected percentage of deaths is 4.3 percent (or 2.4 times the expected death rate from cardiac surgery).[5] Fancy that.

So never trust a stranger (or, in this case, any of the medical centers with their big ad budgets and prima-donna program directors). Do your homework and find out everything you can about a doctor's record. It may be hard to determine if a physician who is new to an institution or a neighborhood is a high-quality one, so I'd go to a physician who has an established record.

As you conduct your search you may be surprised to find that some physicians do not accept insurance. Period. Some of these doctors are indeed very skilled and highly qualified professionals who can afford to take this position (thereby avoiding the hassle of all the forms and the price limitations set by the insurance companies) and feel entitled to earn a seven-figure salary, John Q. Public be damned. Many others with this policy are not so well qualified. Either way, I do not approve of these physicians' shameful way of doing business. Actually, these folks infuriate me. The credo of a physician is to heal the sick, not to take advantage of them by charging outrageous prices, turning those who cannot pay away from the door, and not accepting insurance. Luckily, many of the best doctors are participants of health maintenance organizations (HMOs). Don't believe any rumors to the contrary.

There will almost certainly be times when you are confronted with an urgent medical crisis, though not quite a dire emergency-room visit. Perhaps a member of your family has just been diagnosed with cancer or a neurologic disorder like ALS (Lou Gehrig's disease). In such an instance, it goes without saying that you need to find a compassionate, knowledgeable physician in a hurry. Situations like this are often intensely difficult to manage, particularly if the disorder that you or your loved one has is unlikely, in the long run, to be cured. Stress, panic, denial, a feeling of the walls closing in or of one's worst fears suddenly becoming an inescapable reality—all these mind-numbing emotions converging at once can make for a hellish experience. But one must rally to make sure that logic, coolheaded thinking, and common sense prevail at precisely this most terrible moment.

My suggestion in this case is that you actually see as promptly as you can *not one but two* physicians, both specialists in the field, but one involved in research and the other involved in patient care. This way you will benefit, in theory, from the state-of-the-art knowledge of the former and the highly expert but still hands-on, sympathetic people skills of the latter.

I'll give you an example. A dear friend recently received news that she has ALS—a life-threatening neurologic disorder. When she first began experiencing troubling symptoms she went to see an excellent and compassionate neurologist of sterling reputation. He diagnosed her condition, took all the time needed to explain the ailment to her as carefully as possible, scheduled the tests my friend needed, but also suggested she consult with a physician involved in clinical research just to see what he might have to say about the very latest treatments, state-of-the-art research, etc.

She did see that research clinician, and though his manner was off-putting and somewhat cold, he did at least give her an education about the most current lines of research and treatment. Thus both physicians had their merits, and both visits were worth it. The research doctor, though far too callous as a human being, did have access to the latest study protocols. The real "doctor" took care of the patient.

The problem with many physicians who are involved in research, by the way, is that they sometimes lack the human touch and are often preoccupied with their specific goals: to get funding, to begin and conclude studies, and, yes, to find an answer, or in this case a cure, to a dreadful disease they surely hate with every fiber of their body.

I almost always have my staff help the patient make an appointment for the studies I have suggested, especially when they are complex studies. In addition, my staff always tries to send the patient to a lab that accepts his or her insurance. So if you see a physician, regardless of his status, who ignores you during your interview and simply sends you on your way for exams without helping you, I would suggest you tell him (and his superior) that you are not satisfied with his care.

In the past few years there have been any number of books, magazines, and news articles listing the "best doctors" in this or that field. I am not altogether sure how these lists are compiled, but I have made a point of reading all of them. They are actually rather entertaining, or they would be if this was not such serious business. Some of these physicians have been studying lab animals for years rather than seeing patients. Others are just administrators. My favorite publishers sell their book (I happen to be listed in this one) to the public, but they also do a lively business selling a plaque to every doctor listed in that book for $200.

And how do they sell it? In my case a salesperson dropped it off in my office and told the office manager to either send it back (at our cost) or to send a check. I told him to come pick it up or accept a small fee. It's now hanging on my wall.

In my opinion, the most dangerous such list is the one focusing on the "best" cardiothoracic surgeons, which is compiled by the New York State Department of Health (many states have similar lists, which can usually be obtained on the state's website) every year[6] and published in most of the New York newspapers, including the *New York Times*.

This list ranks cardiothoracic surgeons and the hospital centers in which they work based upon their "operative mortality." There are different patient "risks" (essentially "high-risk patients"—a sick elderly female, for example—versus "low-risk patients"—a healthy young male, for example) placed into an equation to weigh a surgical death, but nevertheless a death is a death. What this has created is something I call the "*New York Times* syndrome." This deadly syndrome actually is responsible for hundreds of deaths in New York State each year.

Let me explain. Three major studies conducted about twenty years ago that compared operative (bypass surgery) to medical treatment (CASS, VA Trial, European Cardiac Society Study) all reached similar conclusions.[7-11] Sicker patients, meaning those with the most disease, have a greater chance of survival when they are operated on rather than treated with medications. Yet the sicker the patient, the more likely he or she is to die during surgery. Self-serving surgeons are thus often confronted with a dilemma: Whether or not to operate on a patient with a 20 percent risk of surgical mortality who has a 50 percent risk of dying anyway within a year and thus risk having their "best surgeon" status tainted by a death on the operating table and then published for everyone to see. (In their defense, surgeons never like to lose patients. And, thanks to the rise of the 1-800 SUE YOUR DOCTOR television ads, they always run the risk of a lawsuit in such cases.)

But here is what often happens as a result of this ridiculous and unintentionally dangerous list. A patient is admitted to the CCU with a large heart attack and recurrent angina (chest pain). The angiogram shows a severely enlarged heart with an ejection fraction (percentage of blood ejected from the heart in a single beat) of 20 percent (normal is 50 percent), and severe triple-vessel disease, including a proximal area of the major (left anterior descending) artery. The patient is also diabetic, female, and seventy-five years of age.

Here's the catch. In my opinion, there are many list-conscious surgeons who would refuse this case because of the significant possibility that the patient might die during or shortly after the operation, even though they are aware that the patient would be more likely to survive with surgery than with just medical therapy. I've interviewed many cardiologists in New York State, and most of them agree with this.

Many surgeons have confided to me other ways in which a senior cardiothoracic or CT surgeon diminishes his mortality data (other than by being a very good surgeon). These tricks include the following: The senior surgeon places his junior surgeon as the primary surgeon on the case and places himself as the *assistant* on the operative report, thus eluding responsibility for the death if the patient expires.

Since only pure bypass surgery is surveyed and tabulated by New York State, and not, for example, surgeries involving valvular disease, it has been suggested to me that some surgeons, as a precaution, will put a few unnecessary stitches in the mitral valve during an operation (so now the patient had valvular surgery as well) and thus escape the burden of a tabulated death, should a high-risk patient die on the table. I know of an even more egregious episode in which a heart surgeon who probably realized that his patient was going to expire and that he was going to have a reportable fatality on his hands went ahead and placed a mechanical aortic valve in the patient possibly to avoid tarnishing his statistical standing. To the best of my knowledge (this was confirmed by several of my colleagues), the patient did not have enough disease present in his aortic valve to justify the replacement.

I am aware of one hospital that was known to transfer patients who were expected to die to its affiliated nursing home next door to avoid a tabulated death. These days, thankfully, all deaths within thirty days of surgery are reported, whereas previously only those patients who died *inside* the hospital were considered operative mortalities.

You may find, therefore, that some of the surgeons boasting the lowest surgical mortality may have in fact caused more deaths than their colleagues because they have turned down cases like the ones mentioned above. Perhaps they even manipulated the thinking of the cardiologist and of the family as well in order to convince them to decline the surgical option. How do they do this? The surgeon tells the family that it is very likely that the operation could lead to (let's say in this case) Mom's death or a devastating stroke. After painting a gruesome picture, he might add, "I'll still go ahead with the operation if you want me to," but he already knows that in 99 cases out of 100 the family will decline the procedure.

This may not be for the faint of heart, but I have known of surgeons who crack open their patient's chest and begin the operation but then decide it's too risky and close the patient up. Many of these surgeons have a very low surgical mortality rate, but at what cost? Can you imagine waking up in pain from surgery and with great apprehension about your prognosis and the course of the healing process only to find out that you had your chest cut open for no reason? Nothing was repaired, and all you have to show for it is a new scar. Needless to say, it would now be impossible to find another surgeon to operate on you not only because a colleague had walked away from trying to save you but because you have a huge, freshly healing scar. Believe me, things like this happen all the time. But there's almost no way of knowing which surgeons do this, and it is almost impossible to report.

It should come as no surprise that there is an unwritten rule among surgeons in most hospitals that says never take a case from another surgeon who refused it because of the high surgical mortality potential. Or in their own words: Don't take on someone else's problem, and above all, don't get dumped on.

To illustrate what I mean here, in the spring of 2003 I did something unheard of among doctors. A cardiothoracic surgeon suggested to a hospitalized patient of mine that coronary bypass surgery was too tricky and risky for him and thus essentially turned him down. Yet after consulting with other cardiologists and another cardiothoracic surgeon I was convinced that the patient needed surgery. The only catch was that it was very difficult to convince another heart surgeon at my hospital to perform the surgery because his colleague had turned the surgery down. So I transferred the patient from Montefiore Medical Center to Columbia Hospital and a team of surgeons who thought the patient would do better (and live longer) with bypass surgery. Not the right thing for me to do politically, but the right thing to do for the patient.

Let's imagine then that there are 1,000 patients turned down every year in New York because they have a likely surgical mortality rate of 20 percent (the average surgical mortality rate in New York state from 1997 to 1999 was about 2 percent and perhaps a one-year mortality of 25 percent). Instead of going to surgery, if these 1,000 patients are treated with medications, their one-year mortality rate may be as high as 50 percent. At the end of one year, then, the *New York Times* syndrome has likely been responsible for the deaths of 250 patients who might have lived longer lives.

Thus it is possibly the case that at least a few of the surgeons who rank at the top of this list, that is, those with the lowest mortality rates, are there because they turn the tough cases away. (Having noted this regrettable fact, I suppose I should concede that if one of these surgeons does agree to perform a procedure on you or on one of your loved ones, then you can take it for granted that you have a low-percentage chance of surgical mortality, which is important.)

Moreover, the list *is* important for two reasons. First, it tells you how many operations a surgeon performed that year. You don't want to let a surgeon near you unless he has performed at least 200 operations in the past year. Second, it tells you which surgeons are to be avoided: those with the very highest surgical mortality. In fact after New York State's bypass-surgery profiling, some of the smallest hospitals with the highest mortality rates closed their bypass programs, thus saving many lives. But these worthwhile contributions are outweighed, I would insist, by what the list does not tell you about the surgeons who simply don't accept the tough cases or about those who perform some sort of valvular surgery on a dying patient to keep that mortality from entering the database. Needless to say, I could name names of surgeons who manipulate the data in order to give themselves a very low surgical mortality.

A few years ago I read a paper published in *The Journal of the American College of Cardiology* (October 1998). In their study, the authors, Eric Peterson, MD, et al., claimed that they "found no evidence that New York's provider profiling limited procedure access in New York's elderly or increased out-of-state transfers."[12] What that means in plain English is that in spite of their higher risks of mortality, the study suggests that high-risk patients in New York were still operated on.

Yet, you did not even need to look at the fine print to learn that this study was conducted on patients who had bypass surgery between the years of 1987 and 1992. However, it is only since 1992 that the New York State Department of Health has released their mortality statistics to the public and thus to the press, and it has taken a few more years for this annual news release to influence patient selection. Thus, only after Dr. Peterson's study was concluded could you find surgeons' mortality rates in the *New York Times*! And so I stand by my claim. Many surgeons won't operate on very high-risk patients if they know those deaths will be published in the local papers.

While we are on the subject of these lists, I have to say I find it hard to trust any of them, unless we are talking about a list of doctors who are guilty of criminal misconduct. You can look this up on the web at *www.fsmb.org*. That site lists each individual state's medical board site. There you can search under professional misconduct to see if your doctor has been listed. You might be surprised by what you find.

Finally, what should you do if you've got no insurance or you have Medicaid? One of the best-kept secrets is that most large hospitals have clinic systems that provide some sort of discounted care to the uninsured or free care for Medicaid patients (since they must accept Medicaid outpatients and in fact get paid quite well for treating them). These centers are staffed by medical residents in training who are often smarter and already better doctors than many of the second-rate doctors out in the community. In addition, all the resident doctors must have an attending physician in the clinic in case they have to consult with him or her. What's more, some of the hospitals even supply discounted medications to clinic patients.

The downside to all of this is that your doctor will not be taking care of you when you are admitted to the hospital. Instead, you will be admitted as a service case, and other residents in training will care for you. But again, if you chose a top-notch hospital, you could end up with better care than if you paid thousands of dollars out of pocket for care in a mediocre community hospital at the other end of town. The clinic is likely to be a bit crowded, and it may be a bit more difficult to get special tests or consultations, but again, the care could end up being quite good. Finally, since residencies only last a few years, you won't have the same doctor for more than three years.

So how do you choose a good doctor? Here is a list of tips I would suggest you follow.

1. Call the physician's office. First, you'll see if the staff picks up the phones in a timely manner, and you'll find out if they are attentive and cordial. The quality of the doctor's staff is often a reflection of the doctor. You can ask the staff where the doctor trained in residency, went to school, and whether he is board certified. Check out the medical school rankings. You can also find out which hospital he admits to. If you're not happy with the staff's response, then you should go on to the next office.

2. Meet and talk to the doctor. Just because you made a trip to the doctor's office or a doctor came to see you at the hospital doesn't mean you're stuck with him. If you're unhappy with his demeanor or mannerisms, if he is unkempt, or if you just don't feel comfortable, then either go see or ask for another doctor. If the office is dirty, walk out before meeting the doctor.

3. Disregard all advertisements.

4. Do not call 800 numbers at the local hospital in your search for a doctor.

5. If you end up in a hospital where your physician does not work, do not automatically accept the physician assigned to you. Have the staff call your doctor and see if he can suggest someone.

6. Only accept someone else's advice about their physician if you feel your friend has done his or her homework.

7. When your doctor sends you to a specialist, always ask him for two different recommendations. Unless you have the greatest trust in your doctor, avoid doctors who rent space from him. Also, avoid the doctor's spouse or a relative of the doctor. (I would ask him if you think that might be the case.)

8. Never wait in an office for more than an hour. You shouldn't feel like you're part of a herd. Having to wait for hours often means your doctor is too cheap to get another partner.

9. Make sure the physician accepts your insurance. Why pay for a service if there is an excellent physician who is in your HMO or insurance plan?

10. If you have no insurance or only have Medicaid, go to a clinic at a university medical center.

CHAPTER 2

How to Survive
Your Hospital Stay

When Henry de Bracton wrote in his book *De Legibus* in the year 1240 that "an ounce of prevention is worth a pound of cure," he coined an adage that could not have been more precise or far-reaching in explaining the importance of preventive medicine. The best way to survive your stay in the hospital is, quite obviously, never to end up there in the first place. But the chronic and endemic abuse of tobacco, alcohol, drugs, and unhealthy food in our country has led to millions upon millions of otherwise preventable hospital admissions and, sadly, to the unnecessary and premature deaths of millions of our fellow human beings. Smokers harm themselves with every puff they take, and the consequences of their habit are too awful, too numerous, and too well known to need review here. Alcohol abuse takes a terrible toll on a variety of organs and systems in the body, and, needless to say, drunken driving (not to mention drunken living) causes tens of thousands of injuries and deaths annually. Drug abuse causes all manner of harm to the body and creates equally dangerous situations on our roads and high-ways. Habitual consumers of fast foods and processed foods are loading the dice against their prospects for physical well-being every day.

I don't want to preach too long from the bully pulpit here, but isn't it obvious that if you abuse your complex hearing apparatus by playing loud music directly into your ear for several hours a day you will eventually go deaf? Or that while aggressive driv-ing might get you to your destination a minute faster, it is much more likely to get you a bed in an emergency room? You must treat your body and mind well if you wish to remain healthy and out of the hospital. Adhere to simple common sense and to the advice a competent physician gives you, and you will prevent many admissions to the hospital.

But since I cannot change human nature, just as I cannot stop the aging process, and because accidents do happen, I choose in-stead to confront the realities of surviving what is in the course of day-to-day living an inevitable experience for most Ameri-cans: a stay in the hospital. In the first part of this chapter, I will focus on the crucial but often overlooked first step for any person facing hospitalization, emergency or not: *Get yourself into a good hospital!* Once you have taken that fundamental first step, I want to describe for you the manifold dangers that are poten-tially in any and every hospital, good or bad, and tell you what you can do about them so that you can leave the hospital in bet-ter health than you were in when you were admitted.

Finding the Right Hospital

Let's consider a few scenarios. Let's say you get pneumonia or are diagnosed with systemic lupus or your congestive heart failure condition has gotten noticeably worse in recent years, and your physician advises a surgical solution. What do you do? Assuming you have a physician you trust and admire, what hospital does he recommend? And why? Are you sure you feel comfortable that his evaluation is based solely on the merits of a given institution? And on the expertise and professionalism of the doctors, nurses, technicians, and administrators there? Or have you ever stopped to think that he may have a good friend on staff somewhere who can really use the business? Or that a given hospital just has a real snazzy marketing department?

It seems that every time you turn on the radio these days you hear about such-and-such university hospital and how it cures diseases that all the other institutions cannot. Everything from wound-care to radiation-therapy, to diabetes, to heart and weight-loss centers, you name it. But that doesn't mean that these centers are truly centers of excellence. In the past hospitals did not pay large sums of money to advertise their services but gained their reputations through state-of-the-art research, highly selective studies published in top-tier medical journals, and just plain good medical practice 24 hours a day, 365 days a year. Believe me, the word got out to the community.

So why do they advertise? Why does any business advertise? Because it is in business to make money. Hospitals are in the business of filling their beds in order to make money. To do so they have large marketing teams willing to spend a great deal of money (millions of dollars in many cases) on advertisements or countless hours coaxing the local or national news networks to put their doctors on the air discussing their expertise. In general, to my sheer dismay, the news networks, even those known for their crack investigative journalists, spend little time investigating the truth about the transparent motives behind this sort of self-promotion.

So, what should you do to set your mind at rest about finding the best hospital in your community? Or, if need be, in the surrounding geographical area or urban center? You should begin by dismissing all the advertisements from your mind. Ignore them completely.

In a perfect world, perhaps the best way to find out which hospital or particular specialty program is truly excellent is to ask a physician you already know as a close friend or relative. Or one known to a close friend or relative. You have to assume that they will give you the unvarnished truth, and that they know their way around all of the major medical institutions in the area. So think hard about whom you know, whom your relatives might know, or whom your best friend down the street might know. Didn't so-and-so's daughter just start her second year of medical school? That kind of thing. It is well worth making a few calls to find out, right?

If that is not possible, and for many folks it is not, I would strongly urge that your first preference as you start your inquiry be to try to find a first-rate *university* hospital and then to seek out the physicians who admit there. You should be willing to travel a considerable distance to do so, too, for after all, your very life could be at stake.

But first things first. Question number one should then be: *Where* is the university whose reputation is being used to sanction and enhance the hospital's reputation and credibility? Is it five minutes away or fifty miles away? More and more these days, in order to survive the cutthroat competition that exists between hospitals for patients, small, less well respected hospitals will shrewdly seek affiliation with larger university hospitals and thus obtain the given university's blessing and glowing reputation without necessarily having the quality doctors, technology, and nursing care to back up that standing. In return, ever mindful of the bottom line, the real university hospital is able to cast its net farther afield and gains access to a greater number of tertiary patients (patients who require special and expensive tests or surgery like cardiac catheterization and bypass) who might otherwise have been sent elsewhere.

I cannot stress enough that many of these smaller "university hospitals" are not *truly* university hospitals; they just use the name given to them by the university hospital as part of "the deal." They are often staffed by less-qualified physicians, and they may not even have residency training programs; or if they do, they frequently have the bottom-of-the-barrel residents. They are more likely than not to be no different and certainly no better than they were prior to the name change.

Here's a classic example of what I mean. Mr. R, a patient of mine for over ten years, got sick while visiting his daughter in a large southeastern city. I spoke with them on the phone and told them to go at once to a university hospital there that I knew had an elite cardiology service. Somehow, though, they ended up at the wrong hospital. The name was deceptively similar, but this place was a small, nonacademic hospital that had only a loose and tenuous affiliation with the real academic center.

They admitted Mr. R with the diagnosis of heart failure and sent him home two days later. The next week he came to my office looking very ill. He showed me his hospital discharge papers and the results of the tests that were performed there. The cardiac echo had been read as normal, but since I knew Mr. R had had a heart attack in the past, this didn't make sense. We performed our own study at once and noticed that almost half of his heart was dead. This "make-believe" academic center's cardiologist had misread his echo. Yet I'm sure that if he had been admitted to the real university hospital (a center where I had in fact studied cardiology), his echo would have been properly analyzed and his treatment would have been correct. So beware of this deceptive and common practice as you begin your search.

Another very useful approach is to do some serious homework on the Internet and at the local library. You might also go to the local university hospital and use their library. (I know that Montefiore's is open to the public.) Once there you can ask the librarian to help you in any number of ways. It is after all his or her job to be knowledgeable about just the sort of information and information links that you are seeking.

For example, if you are suffering from ALS (Lou Gehrig's disease), you could do a thorough search on the Net to find out which facilities are doing the most research on this still incurable disease and what exactly are the credentials and reputations of the doctors affiliated there? You could then call several of the physicians involved in the research and determine which of them, if any, are going to be responsive to your immediate needs.

Or perhaps you just read about the benefits of the new techniques in bypass surgery, like the type they do on a beating heart instead of on a heart-lung machine. What should you do with this information? First, you need to know if what you read is just hype or if it is a real advance in medicine. Contact the hospital in question. Ask to speak to a surgeon, or have your doctor make the call. Almost any surgeon will tell you, if asked, that he or she can do this type of surgery, but the crucial question, of course, is can they do it as expertly as the very best surgeons available? But even the best hospitals and their heavily advertised "best surgeons" may not be all they are cracked up to be, as I noted in the Introduction.

I cannot stress enough the utility of consulting the Internet. Find out what you can about studies in a given area. Where were they done? Which surgeons participated in the study? You can visit a site like *www.acc.org* (the official site of the American College of Cardiology). That is bound to be a big help in a whole variety of ways.

Once you have done this sort of basic research, you need to make some calls to the institution to see if a particular doctor sees patients. I would then do something a bit sneaky. I would call the hospital in the evening and ask to speak to the resident in training on call in that particular medical or surgical field. Ask him to recommend a surgeon for your family. If you happen to know anyone who works in the hospital, cross-check the resident's recommendation, or have him find out if the surgeon is really OK. You would be amazed to learn that many of the department heads or chairmen or chairwomen are not the best doctors, and that many of the doctors who are most commonly written up in the paper or interviewed on the local news channel are in the news because of their narcissism and not their surgical skills. This may sound harsh, but I am not joking. I have no doubt that many of the physicians who read this book will nod and chuckle upon reading this.

Finally, it seems to me that these department heads move around from one hospital (and often one city) to another as often as the star baseball players do today, and in doing so they leave behind any possibility of a binding physician/patient relationship.

You will quickly find that the better hospitals have the most highly competitive residency programs, training programs that are difficult to get into because they only accept the cream of the crop each year from the top medical schools. And that, conversely, the best medical students graduating each spring know which hospitals are the best and so they apply for residency there.

What should be obvious here is one of the plainest and most unavoidable facts of life, namely that not all medical students and not all doctors are made equal. Just as there are brilliant lawyers and decent lawyers and terrible lawyers, or car salesmen, or presidents, or ballplayers, there are some supremely talented doctors, some who are very good, some who are only decent, and some who are pretty awful. It is a scary thought, isn't it? If there is one point I used to make over and over again, it is that you simply cannot make a blind assumption that all doctors, by virtue of the fact that they have an MD at the end of their name, are equally talented, or well trained, or, by their very nature, optimally focused and committed to their given profession and area of expertise.

What I am suggesting is that while it may not be true in every case, it is more than likely that the best American medical school graduates do their training in the best hospitals, the average graduates in the good hospitals, and the bottom-of-the-class graduates in the not-so-good hospitals.

To find out if a particular department at a hospital is very good, I would ask one of the medical residents in the hospital or call up the department chairman's office and ask the secretary, or call up a medical school in the area and speak to the dean's office (they often have some sort of ranking of local hospitals). Rankings by independent magazines like *U.S. News & World Report* may be helpful (*www.usnews.com*), but I would avoid magazines that have special editions dedicated more to advertisements than to the details about their physician or hospital ranking system.

It is also crucial to be reminded that just because hospital A has a great residency training program in cardiology, it doesn't logically follow that they have a great program in pulmonary medicine. Or in the treatment of cancer. And on and on. Never make any assumptions; never give in to a hard sell, or to a soft sell, for that matter. Never take the path of least resistance; never put convenience over seeking out the very best. In the end, you are the only individual who is truly looking out for your best interests. Don't neglect your responsibilities, when so much is at stake.

The Joint Commission on Accreditation of Healthcare Organizations (JCAHO) certifies hospitals on a voluntary basis. According to JCAHO, they perform about 1,500 hospital surveys each year, and they accredit approximately 4,700 hospitals altogether, which represents 92 percent of all U.S. hospitals. Meaning, I suppose, that the remaining 8 percent do not seek or cannot obtain JCAHO accreditation. Needless to say, I would avoid at all costs those hospitals either unwilling to go through the JCAHO process or unable to pass it.[1]

In order to pass this accreditation, charts, medications, hospital policies, etc., are reviewed, and the staff is questioned about patients' rights and medical ethics. To their credit, JCAHO emphasizes the right way to do things and sets standards for appropriate patient care. The vast majority of hospitals receive requirements for improvement, which specify areas of standard noncompliance. They have to address those areas and correct them either through a written plan of correction or at an on-site focus survey. So the process is important for establishing guidelines and quality of care.

But accreditation seems too easy to obtain; there are hardly any real failures. According to Kurt Patton, executive director of Accreditation Services, JCAHO, out of the 1,500 hospitals surveyed each year, only one to three are denied accreditation. So if you see a huge placard in the lobby of the hospital noting JCAHO accreditation, it just means it was one of the 99.9 percent of hospitals that passed inspection.[2]

And you would assume, wouldn't you, that if the hospital is accredited after this arduous process, it must be of the highest quality? Not necessarily. The craziest thing about these visits is that they are announced months in advance. It reminds me of the old World War II prisoner-of-war movies where the camp commandant knew when the Red Cross was coming for inspection. But whereas the POWs were maybe given a new blanket, or a resoled pair of boots, hospitals anticipating a visit from JCAHO are cleaned and painted; stretchers normally blocking passages are put away; nurses are instructed on how to answer questions; and all are told to get to medical records and finish filling out patient charts. One head nurse at a local hospital recently told me that they found several outdated medications in their ICU stock just before their visit from JCAHO. The hospital runs quite well when the JCAHO inspectors arrive.

In defense of JCAHO, I must say that all the hospitals I've worked in take their inspections very seriously, and many an administrator trembles when they think of a JCAHO inspection. I think a senior administrator I recently questioned put this process and its importance in the proper perspective: "Passing may not be difficult, but you get saddled with numerous citations, recommendations, and suggestions, most of which require a written plan of correction with a timetable. To date, our only unannounced survey was a review of how we handled our plan in the months after our last survey. In addition, for the measly sum of $2 anyone can get a transcript of our written report and every violation and recommendation in it. The reporters [he's talking about the press here] have their requests in before the inspection is done. These surveys are anything but a cakewalk; many hospital administrators mark their careers by how many times they have gone through the wringer."[3]

The Emergency Room

Unfortunately, your first encounter with a hospital is very often in the emergency department or, as it is more familiarly known, the emergency room. You may have a broken arm or a bad cut, or you may have burned yourself cooking pasta at the stove. Or your young child may have swallowed some potentially harmful cleaning fluids or prescription medications. However, it is also possible that you may be having a serious heart attack or that you have been badly injured in an automobile accident and are even unconscious or near death. No matter what the situation or how grave it may be, this first encounter you have with a doctor, who is likely a total stranger, is crucial, and one does not have to be watching reruns of *ER* to know that if a mistake is made here it could be most serious. Unfortunately, you or your next of kin will be called upon by the doctor to give your entire history, very possibly while you lie there in terrible pain and terrified about what might be about to happen.

It is therefore essential that you always carry with you a list containing all your pertinent medical data. A sample list might include:

1. your name, phone number, Social Security number, and health insurance carrier ID number;
2. your doctors' telephone numbers/beeper numbers;
3. your illnesses, if any;
4. the medications you are taking;
5. any allergies you might have;

6. your next of kin or who to call in case of emergency, with telephone numbers;
7. and, if you have a heart condition, a copy of your EKG.

Carrying a brief history of your medical problems as well as the medications you take and ones that you are allergic to is particularly important *when you are traveling*. A physician in a strange city far from your home and your personal physician will more often make the correct treatment decision if he or she has your records. A single dose of a medication you are allergic to can lead to shock, possible kidney failure, life-threatening electrolyte abnormalities, or even death.

On your arrival at the ER, I would urge you or a family member (if you are lucky enough to have one there) to insist that the staff member in charge call your regular doctor immediately and that the staff make decisions only after they have spoken to him or her. *Do not accept any excuse.* I would estimate that I am *not* called by ER doctors when one of my patients is admitted there at least half the time. What's more, in my experience there is an even more troubling correlation: The lower the quality of the hospital, the lower the likelihood that I will be called. You would be deeply troubled, even incredulous, at the foolish arrogance possessed by some of the physicians out there. It seems that some of them feel that a simple call to the patient's regular doctor (in my case, the patient's cardiologist) is too bothersome or will be of no real use in that person's care. This defies all logic, of course, and so if you come across such an arrogant physician, or a foolish one, for that matter—and I have met plenty who qualify on one or both counts—tell him he is fired and either transfer out of the hospital or call your doctor and ask him what you should do. Remember you are not only the patient, but also the paying customer.

Not long ago there were no emergency-room specialists, and the doctors who worked in ERs were more often than not those who could not find a job elsewhere, never passed their board exam in internal medicine, wanted to work a part-time job, or just wanted to punch a time clock and not take the responsibility of being on call. Today, however, quality hospitals staff their ERs with board-certified emergency-medicine doctors. The larger university hospitals very often have programs tailored specifically to train these doctors as well.

The emergency doctor is sort of a super general doctor trained to diagnose and triage just about anything. If you are going to go to a hospital for an emergency, this is precisely who you want to see, not some doctor who works in an ER because he or she can't get a job anywhere else. You would be surprised by how poorly staffed some emergency rooms still are.

So what can go wrong in an emergency room? Well, here are a few stories I know about firsthand.

Mr. Brown, an elderly male patient, came to a small community emergency room unconscious. He had a working pacemaker but no documentation for this crucial piece of medical information, so his EKG showed electrical activity that appeared to indicate to the untrained eye of the physician in charge that his heart was beating normally. The pacemaker was working all right, but the patient's heart rhythm was not normal at all. In fact, the rhythm was ventricular fibrillation. That's the potentially deadly heart rhythm that can only be counteracted by an immediate shock with electrical paddles applied to the chest wall. Yet the pacemaker was running at seventy beats per minute and the heart monitor read seventy, so the staff there assumed something else was wrong. The patient's pressure was zero, so they began CPR and called the cardiologist.

Upon his arrival at the ER at 2:00 A.M., the cardiologist looked up at the monitor (the ER nurse yelled to him to do so, thinking all along that the ER doctors might have made a mistake), proclaimed that the patient was in ventricular fibrillation, grabbed the defibrillator, and shocked the patient. Of course by then it was too late to save the patient. The poorly trained, nonboarded doctors in this small ER had failed to notice that the underlying rhythm was ventricular fibrillation—treatable only by a shock—because they had been misled by the pacemaker spikes, which you always see on an EKG when someone has a working pacemaker. The nurses—who knew more ER medicine than the doctors— were just following the chain of command. I would suspect that in a large university hospital the emergency team would have recognized the problem and immediately attempted to shock the patient out of this deadly rhythm. Yet in this small hospital there were only two physicians in the entire emergency room, and neither was board certified. Scary, right?

Here's another cautionary tale. An elderly man, Mr. Green, had collapsed at home and was brought to the local ER, where he was diagnosed as having an acute heart attack. There are several different ways to treat a heart attack now, but in a small hospital the only reasonable alternative is to administer clot-reducing medication. There is no catheterization lab to rush the patient to, and the hospital doesn't perform bypass surgery. The cardiologist arrived within a half hour, just as the doctor in the ER was going to administer the clot-opening medication. He noticed, however, that the patient had a bad bruise over his eye and called the patient's wife in to ask her about it. The wife explained that when her husband collapsed he hit his head on the corner of the marble coffee table. The cardiologist pulled the syringe out of the IV and sent the patient to the university hospital, where he had urgent bypass surgery. Had the patient received the clot-busting medication, he probably would have bled into his brain and died. But luckily for him, and completely by chance, the cardiologist arrived just in the nick of time.

Since this is my specialty, please allow me to digress a bit about heart attacks and the best way to treat them. It no secret now, to the cardiology community anyway, that if you have a heart attack, you want to go immediately to the nearest hospital that can open up the clogged artery. That's because the most recent studies show that opening up the blocked artery with a catheter (an angioplasty or a stent) is much better than attempting to open it with intravenous medication (known as thrombolysis or clot busting). The best hospitals have teams of experts who are available to perform this procedure night and day.

But in the heat of the moment, when lives are often at stake, a great deal of confusion can arise. The first part is quite easy. Never go to a small community hospital if you are having a heart attack. That's because small hospitals usually don't have a catheterization lab where the doctors can open up your artery. Thus, if you suspect you are having a heart attack and the emergency medical technician confirms that you are, make sure you are taken to a hospital that can help you. Do not allow the ambulance crew to take you to their favorite or even the closest hospital if the one that can help you is just a few more minutes away. Even if you have to travel several extra minutes or you must be moved from a small hospital to one with a real catheterization lab, you're still more likely to do better with the invasive approach than with the clot-busting medication.

The tough part is deciding which hospitals have a true 24/7 catheterization lab and which ones just say they do. Many hospitals can open up their lab at any hour and perform an angioplasty, but they often prefer not to (the lab is either slow to get ready or the doctors don't wish to run in in the middle of the night). In reality, it takes a very well-organized lab that has several competent techs and doctors (not just one or two) who can take a call schedule and be ready within the hour. Most labs, however, are not truly ready and willing to do the right thing: take a patient with an acute heart attack to the lab and open up the vessel that is causing it. Thus if you are sent to a hospital that is really not ready and willing, you will get the second-best treatment, a thrombolytic that might open up the clot.

It's basically like having a clogged drain at home. You can call an expert plumber who will bring the snake and open it up, or you can pour some Drāno down the drain and wait for it to open up, if it does. But the analogy stops here, for unlike a drain, the heart and its arteries are living flesh, and the longer it takes to open up the artery and to nourish the heart with blood, the more heart tissue will die. We also know that the bigger the heart attack, the more likely you are going to die from it, either immediately or in the future.

In the practice I share with my partners, if we are called about a patient with a heart attack late at night, we will send the patient to the hospital where he will be treated the fastest—sometimes even to a hospital where we don't have admitting privileges.

While I am on the topic, I'd like to mention the increasing prevalence of mobile heart-catheterization labs (cath labs in a trailer) and caution you against ever using them except in the direst emergencies. A few years ago I was astonished to see mobile cath labs for sale at a cardiology meeting I was attending. Doctors who own this equipment can charge extraordinarily high fees because they can bill for the use of the equipment and for doing the study. In general, the fee for the use of the equipment and the cath lab itself can be as high as $5,000, while the fee for performing the test can be as little as $400. That's quite an extra fee, isn't it?

I can't imagine why anyone would submit to having a dangerous procedure performed in a trailer. *Ever.* Most cardiac procedures done in a trailer are nonemergency diagnostic studies to look for coronary disease. But wouldn't you rather get the study done in a fixed lab that is part of a hospital?

The same problem exists with cath labs located at small hospitals that can't perform heart surgery or even an angioplasty. Why would you submit to a catheterization at a hospital that cannot open up the lesion with a balloon catheter, stent, or bypass surgery? And what if you get sick during the angiogram? Do you really want to be in a hospital where they'll have to call an ambulance and transfer you to another hospital to get the proper care?

More and more, in order to survive in this economic jungle, smaller hospitals are indeed building cath labs, and unfortunately, they are being licensed by their state to perform cardiac studies. I say "unfortunately" because in general these smaller hospitals often allow less-qualified doctors to perform these studies. And since money is the bottom line, the administrators of the hospital often close their eyes to unscrupulous activity if the doctors who are involved are making millions for the hospital. In general, it's easier for bad docs to hide out in places like this.

I know that there are biased nonrandomized studies conducted by and for the purpose of defying this logic (that it is no safer to get this procedure done in a modern large medical center), but I wouldn't believe it.

It is worth pointing out here that I have also seen any number of patients admitted into a hospital, even some of the better ones, who probably should have been sent home instead. In some of these cases, the EKG was hooked up incorrectly, or the patient's anxiety and tremor resulted in an irregular pattern on the EKG. Just recently, a patient was admitted with a diagnosis of an irregular and dangerous heart rate when in fact the irregularity was entirely fictitious. A trained medical eye should have noticed the problem and either dismissed the finding or at the very least asked the technician to repeat the test, thus ending this temporary conundrum.

These mistaken diagnoses happen way too often, resulting in uncalled-for admissions of patients and treatments with unnecessary and potentially quite dangerous medications, not to mention sometimes exorbitant costs to the patient and to our society. In the middle of the night this may sometimes be unavoidable.

But since it is also always best to err on the side of caution, the patient or his next of kin must insist that the ER doc fax the results to the patient's doctor, especially if that physician is a specialist in the field.

As you'll read later, many hospitals also pressure doctors to admit patients. You'll never hear this as part of official hospital policy, of course, but hospital chiefs and administrators have sent the word to their ER docs to "admit as many patients as you can" since hospitals make money when the beds are full.

In general, then, if you have any choice in the matter at all, insist on going to a large university hospital emergency room that has a staff of board-certified emergency-room doctors, and preferably a teaching program, as well. While these emergency rooms may be noisier and more crowded and seemingly chaotic than those of the community hospitals, this is where you want to be if you are really acutely ill. I would strongly urge you to work through any sense of fear or morbid worry such an exercise creates and take the time to find out a bit more about the emergency rooms in hospitals in your community *before you really need to go there,* because if and when the moment comes, you and your loved ones, even your coworkers, etc., should have a clear idea of where you want to be taken.

If you are at home or at the office, or anyplace else where you are still in control of events, and you need to go to the hospital on an emergency basis and have access to a phone or a cell phone, you are within your rights to ask—to insist, really—that the ambulance driver take you precisely where you want to go: to the hospital of your choice. In large urban centers there are often several hospitals located very close by. Many hospitals have purchased their own ambulances to patrol the streets in order to scoop up patients and bring them to their facility. I once witnessed the arrival of four ambulances affiliated with four different hospitals at the scene of a minor car accident. If this happens to you, demand that you be taken to the hospital of your choice, even if the driver expresses some reluctance to do so. It could well save your life, or, at the very least, vastly simplify and improve the quality and outcome of your hospital experience.

But let's say you have fallen ill or been injured seriously, and for whatever reason you have been taken to a hospital emergency room that your physician is not affiliated with or, even worse, you have no primary-care physician to begin with. You now find yourself admitted to a hospital and assigned a doctor you have never met and know nothing about to care for you. You must not ever make an assumption that the doctor in question must be good because he was recommended to you by the hospital. The truth is that being a good doctor may have nothing to do with why you are now that doctor's patient. Many hospitals have rotations where, essentially, the next doctor up in the rotation gets the next patient. Other times the ER physician might be a close friend of the doctor he has assigned to you. Do you want to risk your life on such a gamble? As I have mentioned in another chapter, if you have no other option, the nurses almost always know which doctor is good and which is not, but they are almost always afraid to say anything for fear of slander, lawsuits, loss of job, etc. Even so, it never hurts at least to ask the nurse if there is a doctor that she or he would recommend. If you have no primary-care physician or have not seen a physician in years and thus have no one to call, then you are in no position to benefit from a trusted doctor's guidance in this sort of situation. So, as a word to the wise, I cannot urge you strongly enough to establish and maintain a strong relationship with a qualified doctor.

If you do have a primary-care physician, then make sure the doctors at the hospital call him at once. If one of my patients ends up in a local hospital that I am not affiliated with, in most circumstances I can still be of great help to him. First, I can give a detailed personal medical history to the doctors at the other hospital. Second, I will very often know many of the physicians who are affiliated with that particular hospital and can help the patient choose a doctor to take the best possible care of him while he is there. Finally (see below), if I think the hospital is substandard, for whatever reason (and you would be surprised to know how many hospitals are), I can suggest to the patient and family that he be transported at once to another hospital.

What to Do if You Have Been Taken to a Substandard Hospital

So, let's say you do end up in a small or potentially substandard hospital you know nothing about. You either don't have a relationship with a physician or he or she cannot be reached. What should you do? My usual suggestion is: *Get out.* Many patients naturally are wary of insulting the staff at the hospital, and thus they cross their fingers and stay and hope for the best. Yet I ask, would you go into a used-car dealership and buy a car without knowing anything about it? Are you going to let a bunch of strangers make decisions about your life and allow them to perform surgery on you if you need it? There are bad doctors out there, some performing surgeries for questionable reasons and with less than positive results. As I have written above, many small, nonacademic hospitals are often staffed by physicians who trained in less-well-qualified medical schools or who graduated near the bottom of their class. University hospitals, on the other hand, don't give admitting rights to those physicians who did not pass their board examinations. Yet smaller hospitals—so dependent on filling their beds for their survival—will give admitting privileges to some of the most awful doctors imaginable. Indeed, in my experience, the very busiest physicians (and thus the physicians who generate the greatest number of hospital admissions and total billings) are given carte blanche to do whatever they wish, since the financial well-being of the hospital depends on their admissions. Are you going to put your life in the hands of these people? When many of the doctors who work at these small hospitals would consider no other course than going to major medical centers when *they* need surgery? Do you wonder why? I've seen countless examples of this situation, and it is one of the reasons I decided to write this book.

Here's another situation you may face. Because of new regulations and the downsizing of many residency programs, there are not enough house staff, or doctors in training, to go around in many hospitals. I have pointed out that one of the benefits of going to a teaching hospital is that you always have a doctor in training, and often an intern as well as his senior resident, watching out for you, checking your exam and your blood tests, and making sure all the tests that need to be done have been ordered. However, many hospitals have created what they euphe-mistically call an attending-oriented service (or AOS). I think a recent memo placed at one of the units in a hospital I attend best explains it.

> One unique aspect to AOS is, patients are admitted and fol-lowed daily by their Private Medical Attending and/or Hospitalist. The Plan of Care is developed by the PMD (Primary Medical Doctor) and then implemented by the interdisciplinary team. There are no housestaff (i.e. Resi-dents, interns or Medical Students) to manage these pa-tients. The Physician Assistants' address emergent situations that arise on the unit. The daily management of the patient is done by the PMD.[4]

A much more candid memo to the patient therefore might read as follows:

> If you get admitted to the AOS, no one will check your labs, your exam, or make sure the appropriate tests are being done on a timely basis until your doctor comes by to see you.

So if you are admitted to an AOS service, despite the fact that physically you might be in a university hospital, you are es-sentially being treated as if you are in a community hospital. In general, then, if you hear you are going to an attending-oriented service, refuse, if possible, to go. An exception to this rule could be if you are going to be monitored by highly trained nurse practitioners (NPs) or physician assistants (PAs). These people (if not just out of school) can at times be more helpful to you and your doctor than the medical residents.

So how do you get out? First, try to contact your doctor. If this fails, or if you have no doctor, ask someone in your family or one of your friends to call his or her physician and ask him or her to help you. This might sound strange, but many people have called me with this same thought in mind. And if I know the hospital to be inferior I never hesitate to try to help. Sometimes, when the hospital gets wind of the fact that you (as a patient) have taken this step, an administrator may pay you a visit in your room and tell you in no uncertain terms that the doctor—the primary medical doctor described above—you have is excellent. He might even strongly urge that you should stay in the hospital and even suggest that you may be doing yourself grave harm by even entertaining such a "drastic" step. You've got to realize, however, even though clear thinking may be difficult (as you might be in quite a bit of pain, scared half to death, and/or doped up on drugs), that most administrators in any hospital, large or small, good or bad, are concerned with the bottom-line issue of dollars and cents. It should be perfectly obvious that hospitals with the fewest number of beds could face a significant financial dilemma if patients began transferring out on a regular basis.

I am a cardiologist at both a large teaching hospital and other small community hospitals. Shortly after I began my practice, I was summoned to the administration office of the community hospital because they believed I was transferring too many of my patients to the university hospital. I was even denied privileges at one hospital because, and I quote the representative from the board of doctors: "You are coming to this hospital to take our patients away from us and bring them all to the university hospital."

A few years ago my family and I experienced a situation quite similar to the one I just described. My grandfather called me one day to tell me he was having severe abdominal pain. He lives with my aunt and uncle about an hour away from me. We rushed him to a local hospital, where he was diagnosed with an incarcerated hernia and possibly necrotic (dead) bowel. He had no fever, and his vital signs were stable, but we all understood that he needed to have his situation taken care of before day's end.

The next thing we knew a surgeon approached us to say he was going to operate on my grandfather. We found out that this surgeon had trained at the same small, local hospital and that he had been called by a doctor in the ER. When my mother asked him where he went to school he replied, "Disney World." I guess he was too embarrassed to tell the truth, because he never told us where he went to medical school.

Thus my grandpa, who was eighty-seven at the time and had had coronary bypass surgery five years before, was about to be operated on at this community hospital by a surgeon we knew nothing about, other than the fact that he did not train at a competitive residency program and had a poor sense of humor. In addition, I quickly learned that while the hospital had an ICU, it had no specialized ICU doctors on staff. Thus, if Grandpa got sick in the middle of the night, we would have to trust the nurse to take care of him. The decision for me was easy. I had my grandfather transferred ASAP by ambulance to my hospital to have surgery by someone I knew and trusted.

When I told the surgeon we had decided to transfer Grandpa to the university hospital where I practice, he became quite upset. His ego and his suddenly lighter pocketbook got the best of him. He tried to convince my eighty-seven-year-old grandfather (who was receiving Demerol for his pain) that leaving was the wrong choice. He told him that his family was not looking out for him and that he would have to sign a form acknowledging that he might die on the way to the other hospital. We had Grandpa sign the form, the ambulance arrived at the hospital a few hours later, and Grandpa had the operation performed by physicians I knew were good. Thankfully, everything worked out well.

What your mother might have told you long ago—never put your trust in a stranger—has never been more apt. Why go to a physician who might have graduated from a less than well-respected school at the bottom of his class when quality physicians are also on your insurance plan and it doesn't cost any more? Simply put, if you had the choice to purchase a new Mercedes or a KIA at the same price, which car would you opt for? Well, sad as it may sound, many patients are every day opting for the KIA because they don't even take the time to find out who their doctor is or what his or her background—medical school, training, reputation, etc.—is.

Transition from the ER to Your Hospital Room

So now let's say you have made it to a quality hospital either through the emergency room or directly to a room on a medical or surgical floor. The first person you are likely to see is the nurse, if you are lucky, that is. I say "lucky" because registered nurses are a vanishing breed in many hospitals. LPNs, or licensed practical nurses, who have less schooling and thus are less costly to the hospital, are replacing them. Many hospitals even stoop to having technicians dressed up like nurses taking your vital signs as well.

In my experience, the blood pressure and pulses taken by these pseudoprofessionals are often woefully inaccurate. In some cases, patients were actually getting more medication than they needed (potentially very harmful) for their blood pressure because of inaccurately obtained high readings. Once, in a step-down ICU (a closely monitored hospital bed for patients who are not sick enough to go to an ICU), I could not even find a working manual blood-pressure cuff (instead of an automated one), and I was told by the head nurse that most of them had been lost or stolen. After five minutes of arguing I found one that worked and noted that the automated one had inaccurately read a patient's blood pressure because of the patient's irregular rhythm.

The lesson here is always ask the person who is taking your vital signs to tell you what your vital signs are. Then by all means write them down. If you are concerned that they may be inaccurate, then you should ask your doctor to double-check them.

The next visit might be from a medical student or a resident in training. Often he or she will take your history and examine you. Frankly, in spite of what you might think, this is a very good thing. Although these young men and women may be inexperienced, they tend to be very thorough and might find something that they could bring to the attention of your doctor. One caveat is the drawing of blood and the placement of an intravenous line. I would only allow an experienced nurse or a medical resident to do these procedures. If a student tech or a medical student comes to do this procedure, you should politely tell him or her that you have had bad experiences in the past (infections, etc.) and request someone else to come in.

Placement of intravenous lines can be very dangerous if not done using good, proper, sterile technique. A catheter is placed in the vein, and it is usually left in for up to seventy-two hours. (Recent data and new guidelines issued by the Centers for Disease Control and Prevention suggest that it may be left in for up to four days unless complications such as redness, swelling, or inflammation occur.)[5] If it is placed with dirty technique, not properly cared for, or left in too long, it can result in a dangerous infection. This infection is limited not only to the point of entry on the skin but can also lead directly into the vein (phlebitis) and can even cause bacterial endocarditis (infection of the heart), sepsis (infection in the blood with toxic chemicals), a life-threatening fall in blood pressure, organ failure, and possibly death.

Another type of catheter, called the central venous catheter (CVC), is placed in a major vein, usually in the neck or directly below the clavicle. While this provides important access and can deliver more volume of different medications and fluids to the body, it is also associated with a much greater risk of serious, sometimes life-threatening, infections. In one study, it was estimated that 250,000 cases of CVC-associated infections occur in this country every year, and the attributable mortality is estimated at 12 percent to 25 percent for each infection.[6] In order to reduce the risk of this type of infection I would never allow any doctor to place this type of catheter in your groin (known as the femoral vein) since this area is typically less hygienic. I would also request that a senior medical or surgical resident or physician who specializes in ICU medicine—instead of a medical intern or house doctor—place this type of line. Finally, I would make sure that the area is kept dry and clean to prevent other sources of infection. Too many times I have seen these central catheters uncovered, splattered with patient's secretions, vomitus, or, if placed in the groin, even soiled with urine or feces.

This horrible complication is underreported by the hospitals, thanks no doubt to their reflexive fear of a lawsuit or because it is simply overlooked. Just recently one patient I was consulting on died from this complication, while another had to undergo a prolonged course of antibiotics because of infectious complications from an intravenous line.

To minimize your risk of a life-threatening infection, you must report to the nurse any redness or pain at the site and make sure the intravenous line is cleaned carefully and changed every three to four days. If you are unsatisfied with any of the responses you get from a nurse or a tech, or if there is no response whatsoever, then either call the resident doctor or tell your physician when he or she comes to see you. You should insist that all doctors or nurses wash their hands before they examine you or change your intravenous line or dressings. If a team of ten doctors and medical students comes to your bedside, make sure every single one of them washes his or her hands. You can't imagine how dirty some of these people are or what kind of dangerous resistant organisms were infesting the patient they examined before you. Besides, hospital guidelines require that we wash our hands before and after seeing every patient, though many health professionals do not adhere to this rule. There are many days when I'll bet I wash my hands thirty times or more.

A similar risk occurs with a urinary catheter (also called a Foley catheter). This is a catheter placed into your bladder to remove and also measure the quantity of urine. Studies show that these catheters dramatically increase your chance of getting a dangerous urinary tract infection. In fact urinary catheter–associated infections are the most common cause of infection in hospitals and nursing homes, comprising more than 40 percent of all institutionally acquired infections.[7]

While there are specific published guidelines for placing urinary catheters (because of the potential risk of a dangerous urinary infection),[8] I'm ashamed to say that many hospitals place Foley catheters in their elderly patients just because it makes life easier for the staff. When patients need to go, they just go through the tube rather than call the nurse to assist them to the bathroom.

Ask the staff member why you or your family member is about to receive a urinary catheter and if you are not entirely satisfied with the answer, I would politely ask the nurse if you could speak with the doctor about it before it's placed.

It's unusual for a physician to miss a diagnosis like a heart attack, but an even more serious problem, known as deep-vein thrombosis (DVT), and its consequence, a pulmonary embolism (clot to the lung), remain underdiagnosed in many of our hospitals. In some studies, up to 10 percent of patients who had autopsies were found to have succumbed to a pulmonary embolism. It has been estimated that up to 2 million people develop these clots every year and as many as 200,000 die from them. Thus this preventable illness causes more deaths in the United States in any given year than AIDS, breast cancer, and highway fatalities combined.[9]

This lethal illness might be caused by a long ride in a car or an airplane trip (called economy-class syndrome), heart disease, cancer, pregnancy, estrogen-containing medications, and any trauma, especially those to your lower extremities. It can also result from just lying in your hospital bed. For high-risk patients a single injection of a blood thinner (best given when you are in the emergency room and then daily) can prevent the clot from ever forming. If detected early, before the clot dislodges from the veins in the leg and travels to the lung, it is easily treated with blood thinners. Once it's gone to the lung, you could get very sick, extremely short of breath, and even die.

There are therefore two points to remember here. If you end up in the emergency room with heart failure, pneumonia, a broken leg, or anything that might keep you in a hospital bed, make darn sure to ask your doctor about receiving a shot of a blood thinner (usually heparin or a similar drug called Lovenox). If you ever develop swelling of the legs (especially if only on one side) or sudden shortness of breath, ask the doctor to make sure you don't have a DVT or a pulmonary embolism.

To make this diagnosis you need a smart clinician, some luck (since even the best of us miss this diagnosis sometimes), and then either a nuclear scan of your lungs or a new type of rapid-imaging CAT scan. If you have been admitted to a quality university hospital staffed by competent nuclear-medicine doctors and radiologists, you are probably in luck since these studies are not that simple to read. In one hospital that I know of, the nuclear technician is always on call and will come to the hospital to perform the test on a weekend. Yet, unfortunately, none of the nuclear medicine *doctors* will come in until Monday if called on a Saturday or Sunday. Often a radiology resident, with much less training than the attending physician, is given the task of interpreting the study instead. If the study is done on Friday night, three days may pass at some hospitals before the study is read. The other option, the rapid-imaging CAT scan, must be read by a qualified radiologist.

Don't let this happen to you. If you are the patient, insist that the study be done and read that day. Call the president of the hospital if you need to, but get it done.

So at the risk of repeating myself, always ask your doctor if you are at risk of developing these blood clots. Ask if he or she can put you on medication (usually a blood thinner given by injection) to prevent it. You'd be surprised how many doctors either aren't aware of this protocol or forget to write for it when you're admitted to the hospital. As an extra preventative measure, if you're able to get out of bed, do so regularly and walk around as much as possible.

No matter what study you are going to receive, ask the staff why it's been scheduled, and if it doesn't make sense to you, ask to speak to your doctor before you're wheeled away on a stretcher.

Two years ago my dad had a hip replacement at a rather famous hospital in New York City. At about 10:00 P.M., a few days after the operation, he began complaining of excruciating pain in that area. A house physician assistant was called and an emergent X ray was ordered, only what was requested was an X ray of his knee. My dad argued with the radiology tech as best as he could, but he had been sedated and so the tech ignored him and took the X ray of his knee.

Fortunately for my father, his son is a doctor. I called his orthopedist at home and insisted that he rush to my dad's bedside immediately. A subsequent X ray of his hip showed that his replacement had come out of its socket. Eventually the surgeon was able to manipulate the hip replacement back into place.

Another thing to be on the lookout for as you "police" the situation in your room is the handwritten acronym VSS on your chart. It means *vital signs stable,* but it really means that your doctor probably never bothered to check your vital signs (blood pressure, heart rate, respiratory rate, and temperature). The days of the bedside clipboard are vanishing, and more often today, the person who takes them (more about this later) logs vital signs into a computer. So in order to check or record your blood pressure and heart rate over the past twenty-four hours, your physician must log on to a computer.

Since the institution of computerized vital signs, I have noticed countless occasions when physicians just scrawl VSS on the written progress notes, usually because they did not even check. It takes a couple of minutes to log on and review all the vital signs, but for some doctors that is just too long. I have seen this done by physicians in an ICU, and I once even underlined in disgust the VSS placed by another physician and made mention of it in my note.

To solve this problem I would suggest the following. First write down your vital signs when the tech does them or, if you are very lucky, when a real nurse or doctor does them. When a physician comes to see you again, ask him what your vital signs are. By doing this you will resolve two potential problems. One, if he declines to tell you or tells you some other numbers that don't match up, it is time to get another doctor. Two, it will remind the doctor to check your vital signs. Finally, if you are not sure if the recordings are accurate, kindly ask your doctor to check it himself.

Essentially, a physician's notes should accurately record the vital signs and not mention that they are stable. If anyone reading this book is involved in hospital administration, I suggest you go and look at your records, and you will discover how often this is occurring at your hospital.

Getting the Right Medications

You're in the hospital, you have a nice, clean intravenous catheter in your arm, your vital signs are accurate, and it is time for you to get your medication. Here again there are risks. Are you going to get the correct medication? For the most part, you probably are. However, do not be fooled by the statistics a hospital may publish about reported errors in medication. As chilling as it must be to read this, I have to tell you that, for the most part, medication errors are not reported. Instead, someone realizes the error, discontinues the drug, and prescribes something else, essentially employing the no harm/no foul philosophy. Here's what I mean. A patient with a history of heart failure is receiving too much intravenous fluid and may develop fluid in the lungs. The doctor is called, notices the error, gives the patient a potent diuretic, and everything is fine. (Sometimes, however, a patient in a similar fix will end up on a ventilator in an intensive care unit because the nurse never bothered to look in on him.) These episodes are much more common at night, when nurses often take extended sleeping breaks and the medical residents (most of whom are overworked) are less likely to take an extra look at the patient. Many of the medical residents reading this might nod their heads in agreement, while the hospital board members might be shaking theirs in impassioned opposition.

To diminish this sort of risk, you or a family member should always carry a list of medications you are taking at home as well as one for those medications that may be dangerous for you to take. Make sure that the nurse and doctor who admit you review the medications you will be receiving in the hospital with you and your primary-care physician. Make sure you notify the staff when you last took these medications and make sure you don't miss a dose. In my experience, patients who are receiving treatment or, worse, waiting to receive treatment in our emergency rooms don't receive all the medications they might be scheduled to take if they were home; it is just something often overlooked by the staff. I mentioned this previously, but it bears repeating here: You should also always carry a list of your medical problems, or even a recent copy of your office visit with your doctor.

If you are undergoing an extended hospitalization, I would ask a family member to call you before you go to bed and ask you how you feel, how your breathing is, and if you have any discomfort anywhere in your body. If you do, call the nurse and ask her to call the doctor. Unfortunately, in my experience, some nurses may just ignore your request, so call back in a half hour and ask what's going on. If you have the financial means, by all means hire one of the day nurses (or technicians) to stay with you for the first few nights following surgery or admission to the hospital. The medical resident physicians usually know who is qualified, and thus I suggest you ask them if any of the staff moonlights for private duty. Stay away from agencies that will provide you with just about anyone, no matter how unqualified, uncaring, or sleepy—just ask poor Andy Warhol.

For example, I recently paid a hospital technician $21 an hour to watch over my grandfather for the 11:00 P.M. to 7:00 A.M. shift. She helped him to the bathroom several times a night (since we made sure the urinary catheter was out) and gave him a sponge bath in the morning before she left. He felt pampered, and I think it really lifted his spirits.

Transportation Inside the Hospital

As you surely know from television show, if not from firsthand experience, patients are routinely transported throughout the mazelike corridors of a hospital—very often like cattle, in my view—for important tests or examinations. Often they are told not to eat until the test is over, and sometimes, because of the inevitable delays, they must wait without eating until nighttime. So bad things can happen when a staff person who does nothing more than push a stretcher around the building wheels off an elderly confused patient who has been sedated on an empty stomach. If you become short of breath or stop breathing, the person pushing the stretcher might be the only one standing between you and death.

Once you reach your destination, you might have to wait parked on the stretcher for an hour or so or until it is your turn for the study. If you are thirsty, it's unlikely that anyone will get you a drink. If you have to use the bathroom, you'll be lucky if you're offered a bedpan and a shower curtain to provide you with even the slightest shred of privacy. Once you are done with the test, you must then wait for someone to come along and wheel you back to your room.

Even in the best of hands, patients get sick or die while being transported from a medical bed or even an intensive-care-unit bed. In a widely read text about ICU medicine, an entire chapter is devoted to the transport of critically ill patients. And in this chapter the authors, who are specialists in ICU medicine, note that "no one can ignore the risks of transporting critically ill patients." They then go on to say: "Indeed, all experienced intensivists can recall having grappled with a patient's sudden decompensation in some awkward corner of the hospital."[10]

In a recent discussion with an administrator at a large university hospital, I learned about one death and another near death that occurred during the transport of a patient. These catastrophes were the result of a number of errors, but they might have been prevented if the patients had not been on a stretcher being transported from their hospital bed to the X-ray department. From what I was told, the doctors on the floor had incorrectly administered too much of a sedative to both patients (to calm them down) before sending them for an X ray. In both instances, an untrained transporter (in general transporters in hospitals have no training in patient care) then took the patient to the radiology department. Somewhere on the way, the patients stopped breathing and had a respiratory arrest.[11]

The week I wrote this chapter I had firsthand experience with the transportation of a patient that might have resulted in her death. I was called to see a patient who was admitted to the hospital from the emergency room on a Saturday. According to her doctor, she was a demented woman who came in with some signs of heart failure. She was given some diuretics and oxygen in the ER and was then sent up to the floor around 11:00 A.M., so when I went to see her about noon I expected to find her in her bed. When I got to the floor, I saw her still lying on the transport stretcher outside her room. Though she was hooked up to a small oxygen tank, she was in fact looking quite blue. As scary as it sounds, her oxygen tank had run out. It was empty. Either the transport team dropped her off without telling the medical staff she was there, or the nursing staff just didn't go and see the patient straightaway, as they should have.

I called for the nurse to come immediately with a fresh oxygen tank before the patient died. Thankfully, her color improved with the fresh oxygen supply, but I'm quite sure that had I not come by to see her when I did, the staff doctor would have filled out her death certificate later on that day.

It's hard to estimate how many of these episodes occur in hospitals every day, but my suspicion is that thousands of such events or deaths occur during that precarious time when a patient is being transported to and from his or her bed. So with this in mind I would strongly suggest you have someone with you when you do go for a study, just to make sure you are going to be watched over at all times. And if you are told that Mom or Dad is going to be admitted from the ER into a hospital room and that things are OK now, don't go home until you see that he or she is safely installed in a hospital bed and after you've met the nurse and the house doctor.

Lousy, Dangerous Food

OK. So the food stinks, the place is noisy, your roommate is demented and up all night, someone is sobbing down the hall, the nurses don't always come right away when you page them, and the air feels thick and poisonous . . . you must be in a hospital! You come to a hospital to get better, right? And you probably would feel better if you had some soothing music, a private room, and something tasty to eat. But you quickly learn the hard way that the commercials you've seen on television about your local hospital have been illusory, nothing but a grim charade. You are never going to be the catered-to customer you might have imagined.

In reality, most hospitals are fighting for their financial lives and thus are cutting back drastically and across the board on their services. At the university hospital where I consult they now offer patients a one-choice meal. And they actually call it just that. In other words, you have no choice in ordering what type of food you want. Yes, they usually send around huge snack carts stocked with all sorts of goodies and sandwiches from which patients can purchase items from out of their own pocket. But the hospital will still charge you dearly for that meal you skipped, and of course there is no labeling of sodium or fat content on the food sold as an extra from the cart. Much of it is, in fact, loaded with salt and fat, and sure enough, I have seen countless occasions where sick, elderly cardiac patients are purchasing and eating foods they should not be within a country mile of.

The irony of these cutbacks in areas like food service is that the senior administrators of these hospitals continue to take huge pay raises. Spencer Forman at Montefiore Medical Center, for example, managed to take home over $300,000 more in 2000 than in 1999. His total compensation in 2000 came to $1.6 million.

And while I'm on the subject of food, let's not forget that the wrong food can be as dangerous as the wrong medicine. And not only the obvious stuff, like the high-salt diet for the patient with heart failure or the sugar-laden meal for the diabetic. Incredibly, this sort of thing does happen, but there are other less obvious but no less dangerous ways the food in the hospital can kill you.

Recently a patient my partners and I consulted on was restarted on his blood thinner—Coumadin (warfarin)—after an episode of bleeding that resolved itself. But in spite of days of therapy with Coumadin, the patient's INR level (we routinely check to see if the blood is thinned to a standard protocol) mysteriously did not increase. It happened that the next time I saw the patient he was eating his hospital-prepared lunch. Mystery solved. For there on his plate was a huge serving of spinach. Spinach contains a very high amount of vitamin K, which counteracts the effects of Coumadin.

You would think in a hospital that has a state-of-the-art computerized ordering system for its meals and medications, as well as full-time dieticians and nurses, that something like this wouldn't occur. By happenstance I saw it with my own eyes.

Nighttime in the Ward—Beware

Nighttime, as I mentioned in passing above, is not as safe as daytime. Not on the streets and highways, and certainly not in the hospital. It is an open secret among health-care workers that patients are frequently ignored during the night. Patients ring the call bell in vain for ten minutes and eventually get up on their own only to fall on the floor and hurt themselves; intravenous fluids run dry because the staff has forgotten to change the bag; catheters fall out of patients' veins, leaving trails of blood; and yes, patients stop breathing because no one noticed they were very sick a few hours before. Strangely, in spite of certain obvious disadvantages when it comes to privacy, you might be better off in a room with two beds and on a type of buddy system, that is, if your roommate does not keep you up all night. Needless to say, the best solution, if you have the money and you are ill enough to be genuinely concerned, is to have a private-duty nurse with you at night, unless she falls asleep as well. I have given patients' families the names of nurse's aides that I know and trust who watch over their family members at night, and I can tell you even I have slept better knowing they were there.

The Intensive Care Unit

I think the greatest troubles occur at the hospital—and doubly so at night—after a patient has been transferred out of the intensive care unit (ICU). In the ICU each nurse takes care of only one or two patients, yet when one of those patients gets to a floor bed he or she may be one of as many as ten patients being cared for by a single nurse. In addition, the nurses on the regular floor are usually not really qualified to recognize sudden changes in condition or to care for really sick people. Thus on Monday you might be hooked up to all sorts of monitors and watched over by a specialized nurse, but on Tuesday you could end up seeing your nurse no more than four times in the entire day. And at night, as we know, all bets are off. You might see a nurse only once or twice during the entire night. Get ill sometime in between, while the clerk who is supposed to answer the bell goes on break, and you can see how bad things happen.

If you do not feel well, then tell your doctor you would like to stay in the ICU an extra day. If you are upset with the nursing staff on the regular floor, the best thing to do is to call the hospital president's or medical director's office. Don't complain to the nurse in question or even to her supervisor. Just call up the president of the hospital and politely make a complaint. I would even consider having it typed up and faxed to his office. In my experience, this is about the only way you are ever going to get anything done. Too bad if you hurt someone's feelings. It is your life and your well-being that are at stake. Even at this time, when you are most in need of help, you or those you love must hold each and every medical professional to the highest possible standards. And remember, your hospital care may end up being superb, particularly if you choose your hospital well.

Just as you may be told you need to leave the ICU bed before you think you are ready, your condition may worsen while you are in a regular medical bed to the point where you require immediate intensive care. But in this instance, you may be told that there are no beds available in the ICU and that you must remain in a regular—and unmonitored—bed. Beds in the ICU are of course finite in number and thus can become quite precious when there are lots of sick people in the hospital. Sometimes the ICU staff needs a little urging by your doctor and the hospital administration to get you into their unit.

Thus, it is imperative in such a case that you act quickly and forcefully. Call the hospital administrator at once and document your complaints. The patients and the families of patients that make the call, adamantly challenge the staff to do the right thing, and document the potential dangers in their care are more often than not the ones that get what they want. Good manners, dignity, and trust in the system all sound noble, but I caution you, do not expect to be rewarded for such behavior in many hospitals today.

Here's what you should say. Tell the administrator that your dad (for example) is very sick, that you know for a fact that many of the administrator's own medical staff have suggested to you that he would best be treated in an ICU. But because there is no bed available, your dad may have to be sent to a less intensively monitored bed and possibly suffer the consequences. You have never been a pushy or argumentative person, but when your dad's life is on the line you feel it is necessary to go on record that you have called the president's office (mention the administrator's name) and that you will hold him and the hospital responsible if anything should happen to your father.

I am an unusually hard-nosed doctor, as you may know by now. When I was told recently that there was no room in the ICU for a very sick patient of mine, I called a senior administrator and suggested to her that if my patient did not get a special bed within the next few hours I would make a call to our local congressman's office. Amazingly, a bed was soon made available for my patient.

Here is another true story that illustrates many of the things that can go wrong in a hospital and, in particular, shows what can happen if a patient's true condition goes unrecognized and uncared for.

Mr. C, an elderly patient with diabetes, came to the hospital with markedly elevated sugars. During his treatment in the hospital, he was also diagnosed with cancer of the colon, not an emergency but something that would certainly require surgery.

His medical doctor neglected to call in a cardiologist or at least order a stress test to see if the patient's heart could withstand the stress of surgery.

The night after surgery Mr. C developed chest pain, very low blood pressure, and a rapid heart rate. Believe it or not the patient was being cared for by a dentist, rotating on a surgical service, in what is called a surgical step-down unit, which is essentially a hospital bed with a monitor, a higher nurse-to-patient ratio, and a bed controlled by the ICU team. Calls to an ICU attending that night resulted in orders given over the phone for medications that in retrospect did more harm than good.

It was not until the next morning, on a weekend, that a cardiologist was called to see Mr. C. The cardiologist was able to locate a sonogram machine and found the patient's heart to be severely damaged. He could not say when most of the damage had occurred, but he immediately called the ICU attending who had made the incorrect phone orders the previous evening. Instead of running to see the patient, apologizing for her mistake, and immediately accepting the patient to the ICU for special monitoring and treatment, this ICU doctor attempted to refuse the patient. In fact, from her cell phone—she never did come in to see the patient—she suggested that the patient go to a cardiac floor rather than her special unit, which was geared for sick post-op surgical patients, and thus called a surgical ICU.

Mr. C died that night. I strongly suspect that if the patient had received the correct medications from the ICU doctor, if there had been no delay in ICU care (perhaps if the patient had been sent to the ICU right after his operation, he would have been treated differently), and if the stress test had been performed prior to the patient's surgery, the outcome might have been very different and far less tragic. I was told that the ICU attending was reprimanded, yet nothing was reported to the state. I'm sure the family of the patient was never informed that their loved one's treatment had been so inept, uncaring, and unprofessional. I was recently informed that the family's attorney has filed a malpractice suit against the hospital and some of the physicians involved.

Hospital Staff

It is perhaps a less than well kept secret that even some of the better hospitals in big cities like New York are frequently forced to employ the otherwise unemployable. These untrained people— some of whom seem to be unhappy in their work and in their lives—who admittedly perform some of the most menial and unrewarding tasks in a hospital setting, are nevertheless capable of undermining the whole scheme of providing quality medical care. All of the nurses and physicians I work with—and who will no doubt read these pages—will agree that it is very diffi- cult to get competent help in many areas of health care. I am talking about the little things here. Like a physician answering his page only to have the phone ring for ten minutes—or until he gives up—because the ward clerk is on the phone with her friend or is taking an unscheduled break without informing anyone. This happens all the time at the hospitals where I work, and it leaves me with a bad feeling most days. Soap dispensers not filled with soap, rooms not well cleaned during a patient's stay or between patient stays, blood samples lost or never drawn to begin with, orderlies out on the sidewalk on cigarette breaks when there is crucial work to be done upstairs, medical notes written down on the wrong patient's chart, cold, congealed meals left in front of patients too ill to feed themselves. I don't know what the answer to the problem is, but I do know that it is almost impossible to get fired for performing one of these jobs poorly. It creates a lot of tension and, frankly, a lot of despair for the rest of the health-care team, especially those many beautiful people who do work hard as orderlies, clerks, and transporters yet receive the same pay as those who undermine the system.

Sometimes a little gift from a patient—perhaps a couple of fresh pizzas for the floor—can boost the morale of an otherwise depressed team of health-care workers, and as hard as it is to say this, such an act of generosity may have an impact on the quality of the care you receive.

Being Pushed Out of Your Hospital Too Soon

Many patients often complain that doctors and the hospitals they work for are asking them to leave before they are ready to go. Perhaps you have had this experience yourself. I think you might be right.

Years ago, a hospital or a doctor received payment from your insurance company for each day you were in the hospital. Frankly, this method of billing created an obvious incentive to keep the patient in the hospital for prolonged stays. Keep the beds full, and the hospital makes more money. Insurers could not continue to cover such inflated costs—especially Medicare—and thus they developed a new arrangement based on a code system called DRG (diagnoses-related group).

Essentially, every diagnosis possible is matched to a code, and that code signifies the dollar amount on which the insurers base their reimbursement. There are special agents (usually people who were the top-notch nurses in the past) who review your chart in an attempt to create the highest billing code that will match one of your diagnoses. The hospital is then reimbursed an amount of money based on this code, regardless of whether you stay two days or ten days. Thus, the shorter your hospital stay, the more profitable your admission is for the hospital. Each special agent carries with them a loose-leaf binder containing the DRG codes, how much the hospital is reimbursed for each code, and the maximum number of days that payment will provide for until the predetermined break-even point is reached. Once a patient reaches that point, he or she becomes a financial liability for the hospital, and I will tell you plainly, bottom-line, the hospital's financial liabilities are many times more important to them than your health.

Not long ago I was able to obtain a confidential scale of expected revenue from a major medical institution based on DRG diagnoses. With the scale in hand, I will use a simple case to explain how hospitals can make millions by tweaking the diagnoses of their patients.

Mr. A was admitted to the hospital with chest pain. He had some mild shortness of breath, and although there were no other signs of heart failure, the doctors gave him some oxygen and a diuretic just in case. One of the several blood tests looking for damage to the heart came back mildly abnormal—most likely a lab error—since all the others were normal. He had a two-day stay in the hospital and was sent home for an outpatient stress test.

His doctor's diagnosis and plan was to exclude angina, a symptom of coronary artery disease. Based on the doctor's diagnosis, a DRG number associated with angina pectoris was given. According to this DRG code, the hospital could expect $5,221 in estimated revenue. The physician came back the next day to find stuck to the chart (these are removed after the patient is discharged) notes suggesting that he could consider this event a small heart attack and that he might possibly address the treatment of the patient's heart failure in the emergency room. If the doctor did address these issues in the chart, then the DRG code would be upgraded to acute myocardial infarction with cardiovascular compromise/discharged alive. All that means is that the patient had a heart attack, it was complicated by some heart failure, and he went home alive. For those few changes the hospital's expected revenue would have been $15,731!

The hospitals also have groups of experts whose job is to facilitate your hospital discharge or, in other words, get you out of there as fast as possible. These people might harass your doctor, you, or your family in order to get you out of the hospital as quickly as possible. They often work with the social workers and meet every day in closed rooms to discuss your progress and when and/or how quickly you should be discharged.

In their defense, this strategy can often be quite helpful to you as well. Sometimes it is important to notify a rehab center about patients who will be discharged shortly and will be in need of intensive rehabilitation. Prior to these DRG regulations, there was little incentive for the hospital, or the doctor, to discharge you. Patients waited for days on end to receive the results of simple studies that should have been done in only a day or two at the most. Moreover, it is not always a bad idea to leave the hospital a day earlier than you thought you were going to leave. After all, the food stinks, it is hard to get a good night's sleep, and there are terrible bacteria all around the hospital. You must trust your physician with this important decision. However, if you are sure you need an extra day, most caring doctors will let you stay the extra day, even though the discharge nurse might yell at them.

Still, there are plenty of other occasions, for example, in the case of very sick patients who are old and have less of a chance of fully recovering, when the hospital discharge machine might try to send the patient out to the nursing home too soon. I write more about such a case in the Conclusion of this book.

When you *do* get discharged, make sure your doctor has reviewed your hospital course with you and has gone over all the medications you might be prescribed at discharge. Too often, your doctor will leave you to review all this information with the nurse, even forget to write your prescription. So make sure your doctor hands you your prescriptions before saying good-bye, and make sure you understand everything he or she says.

Not all of us are lucky enough to be discharged straight to our homes. Some patients will be sent to a rehab center for a few weeks to recuperate thoroughly. Occasionally, the "rehab center" will be a floor at a nursing home. If you are sent to such a place, I'd suggest that you not go. At the risk of sounding both harsh and judgmental, in my experience some of the doctors who work at these places are unscrupulous, incompetent physicians who use this work to augment their income. There are doctors who run from one of these nursing homes to the next, doing cursory exams, ordering unnecessary consultations for their buddies to perform, and sometimes making money off of what I call the living dead (elderly, less than fully competent people who long ago lost the opportunity to die with some dignity). In any event, if you need to go to a rehab center, make sure it is just that—a rehab center. And if you have learned anything from this chapter, by all means, when you get there, make sure that the doctor who is admitting you has the decency to call your physician to discuss your case. I would say that well over half the time the doctors at these centers fail to call me. Sometimes they even change the medical regimen we have prescribed for the patient.

If you do become ill in a nursing home or rehab center, you should insist that the staff call your physician immediately. And if they need to send you to the hospital, make sure it is the one you want to go to. Nursing homes have all sorts of deals with hospitals. Nothing written down of course. But both places need to fill their beds, and both appreciate getting patients from each other. In addition, many nursing homes have their own group of specialists who come to see patients at the home. The nursing home prefers to have the doctors see you there, not because it is more convenient for you but because the nursing home is responsible for paying for the transportation.

Again, if you become ill in a nursing home or rehab center and you have a family member who is up to it and you trust your regular physician, insist that you be taken to his or her office. In general, the doctors who make their livelihood doing consults at nursing homes are not the cream of the crop.

If you have a family member suffering from Alzheimer's or some other form of dementia living out his or her dying days at a home, do not allow the home to perform any tests or call any specialists in without consulting you. Scary as this sounds, there are many doctors making handsome livings off of demented and dying patients. Portable sonogram companies may come and scan their bodies, gastroenterologists might perform a colonoscopy because Grandma had some microscopic blood cells in her stool, X rays are done, and surgical procedures are even performed for an old hernia, all for patients who do not need such care. I know this because I've seen it done.

And, finally, if you are admitted to a nursing home, don't count on receiving the same medications you were just prescribed by your doctor as you left the hospital. Nursing homes are usually allowed to spend no more than $250 per day to care for you, and that sum includes *all* your medications. Thus they've conveniently created a "no list," a list of drugs that they don't wish their doctors to prescribe because they're too darn expensive, even if they are far and away the most effective medications for your condition. And if a doctor prescribes a "no list" medication, he usually gets called—or, more accurately stated, harassed—by the nursing-home pharmacy and then ultimately by the home's medical director.

Now, in defense of the nursing home, and as I have taken great pains to make abundantly clear, it is often the case that less-expensive medications are just as good as the more expensive ones. But in certain situations, changes in medications can result in catastrophic consequences.

I've had to contend with these dangerous changes in the medication prescribed for many of my chronically ill but stable heart-disease patients, changes that are made by nursing-home physicians who never bothered to consult with me or my patient. So I suggest that any patient making the transition from a hospital to a nursing home should make sure to continue on the same medications your real doctor has prescribed for you or, at the very least, to insist that the staff at a nursing or rehab facility call your doctor whenever they consider changing any of your medications.

A Week in the Life

To give you a better sense of how prevalent the problems and dangers in most hospitals are—even those that I call university hospitals—I want to capture for you one week's worth of the most serious and daunting issues I have encountered.

I chose the week of March 24, 2003, with no foreknowledge of what might happen and to whom.

Mrs. Blue, an elderly woman, came to the hospital after falling down and fracturing her hip. She was in the hospital for about two days before undergoing surgery to repair her hip. A cardiac sonogram was done, and though she had a murmur, her heart was in good shape. In spite of my recommendation, the surgeons in charge of the case did not put her on a blood thinner before she went for surgery.

The night after her operation, Mrs. Blue became acutely short of breath and developed chest pain and a rapid heart and breathing rate. In addition, her blood-oxygen levels fell. In spite of these symptoms, her cardiogram did not show changes consistent with a heart attack, and her exam did not suggest that she had developed any heart failure.

By now you might have guessed that Mrs. Blue had a pulmonary embolism, right? But neither a physician's assistant nor the orthopedic resident had any idea, so they called the ICU doctor who, by chance, was the same ICU physician I have written about elsewhere in this book. She discussed the case over the phone and unfortunately once again missed the diagnosis. Mrs. Blue was so sick that she was sent to a step-down ICU bed for observation, but despite this, no blood thinner was given to her to prevent further clots and no tests were ordered to finalize the diagnosis.

At 8:00 A.M. the next day, Mrs. Blue was still sick. Her heart rate remained at about 120 beats per minute, and she was still very short of breath. At this juncture, I was paged on the hospital loudspeaker. I was not in the hospital; I was, however, in my car, on the way to the hospital, with my phone and beeper activated. Had they even called my service, I would have answered, but not being in the hospital, I could not hear or answer their page. The PA thus wrote a note at the time: "Patient remains very ill. Dr. Levine paged, but he did not return his call." Talk about setting me up for a lawsuit!

In addition to all this, no one called Mrs. Blue's family to tell them that Mom had gotten very sick, so they were shocked to find out, when they arrived for a visit, that she had been moved to an intensive care bed.

At about 10:00 A.M., after seeing my cardiac patients, I went by to see how Mrs. Blue was feeling after her operation. That is when I heard that she had been transferred to a monitored ICU bed. The staff told me what had happened. I told them, "She has a pulmonary embolism. Did you start treatment or order a scan of her lungs?" In fact, nothing had been done. When I saw the patient in the ICU there was no working intravenous line, and they had not even done a simple chest X ray. And to make matters worse, in spite of the uproar I was creating, there was no ICU doctor or even a nurse there to help take care of the patient when I told them that she had a life-threatening embolism. Just one overwhelmed PA. After a few frantic calls we got the blood thinner started, ordered the special CAT scan of the chest (which showed positive for a pulmonary embolism), and with a tincture of time, medicine, and some luck, Mrs. Blue recovered.

The same day I saw Mr. White, an elderly gentleman who had cancer and who had also suffered a large heart attack after his surgery. I noticed in his records that he had been admitted to the hospital not too long ago for chest pain, but he had never been given a stress test. Someone else might have noticed this and seen to it that he undergo a stress test prior to surgery, but no one had bothered, and now this was water under the bridge. I wasn't involved at that time, so I'll stick to the problems with his care that I saw with my own eyes.

After his heart attack, Mr. White underwent a cardiac catheterization (which confirmed a fairly big heart attack but, luckily for him, showed the other vessels to be OK). He remained quite sick, though, and in particular began to complain of severe shortness of breath and wheezing, mostly at night. His chest X ray showed heart failure. I therefore suggested that he be treated with a potent diuretic, particularly in the evening. The ICU doctor disagreed, suspecting that Mr. White had asthma, and so he gave Mr. White huge doses of steroids in order to clear up his wheezing. Steroids, however, as I told the staff, are known to prevent the heart from healing after a large heart attack and, if administered, in this case, could lead to the death of the patient. I also asked why the patient would have asthma now when he had never had it before and reminded them that heart failure—which he did have—could explain the wheezing and shortness of breath. Against my judgment and, frankly, common sense, they administered the steroids. I was so upset the next day that I wrote precisely that in the chart: *Against my judgment and at potential great risk to the patient, the ICU staff is ordering large doses of steroids.* With that statement in the chart and with my suggestions that they were endangering the patient still ringing in their ears, the steroids were stopped, medications were given for heart failure, and the patient happily got better. His cardiologist, however, needed a few antacids after this battle.

An elderly Miss Blonde was admitted to a community hospital after accidentally taking a bottle of cardiac medications known as calcium channel blockers. Lucky for her she had a pacemaker, which kept her heart beating. In any event I was called to help with her care, along with an internist and a nephrologist. During the night I reviewed the poison-control suggestions via the Internet and then decided to treat the patient with high doses of calcium. The drug worked well, and her blood pressure responded, rising from a low of 60 systolic up to 100. We were also able to decrease the other potent medicines she was on to keep her blood pressure elevated.

Things went well until the evening of the next day, when I was called because Miss Blonde's blood pressure had fallen. I asked if her treatment had been changed in any way. The nurse told me that the nephrologist had given the patient intravenous fluids followed by a potent diuretic called Lasix to increase her urine output.

That combination of medications is also the best way of lowering your blood-calcium level. Thus, I was treating the patient for her medication overdose while this nephrologist was giving her treatment that would ultimately counteract what I was striving to achieve: a higher blood-calcium level. So in order to get the patient's blood pressure back up I had to increase the calcium infusions and stop the Lasix and fluid infusion.

The next day, when I confronted the nephrologist, he told me that no one ever told him the patient had taken an overdose of calcium blockers and thus he was not to blame. Not only had this physician corrupted the patient's treatment by not taking the time to find out the full story behind her illness, he had the gall not to accept any blame or responsibility for what he had done. Thankfully I realized the problem, administered additional calcium, and the patient's blood pressure was restored to a normal level. Within a few days, with the dangerous overdose all but out of her system, she was out of the ICU and feeling much better.

Mr. Baker was admitted to the hospital with a very rapid heart rate. We placed him on medications and took care of that problem. This was the first time we had ever seen him, but he looked chronically ill and admitted that he drank too much. A workup revealed that he had an inflamed liver and chronic hepatitis, and a possible liver mass was detected on a sonogram. An MRI was ordered to see whether or not he had liver cancer. Two days went by and the MRI had not been done, so on the suggestion of the nurses I agreed to discharge him for an outpatient study; after all, the radiology department told us that the study would be done by tomorrow. But when we called to tell the MRI department that the patient would come from home for the study, we were told that made things very different. According to them, Mr. Baker would now have to be scheduled under the outpatient scheduling system, and the next available appointment was in June. Now how do you tell a patient not only that he might have a liver tumor that could probably kill him in six months but that the test to determine if he did have it would not be done for three months? I tried to keep the patient in the hospital and cancel his discharge, but he refused to stay and essentially stormed out. I never saw him again.

Mr. Buchanan is a patient with both severe heart and lung disease. He had a prolonged admission at our hospital and was cared for by specialists in cardiology (me) and pulmonary medicine. He was then discharged on a very complicated medical regimen to a rehab/nursing facility. Two days after his discharge he was brought back to the hospital with severe shortness of breath. When I reviewed the notes at the nursing home I saw that the doctor who was caring for Mr. Buchanan (someone who is a specialist in neither cardiology nor pulmonary medicine) had changed most of our medications for ones he preferred. Mr.

Buchanan eventually was transferred to another rehab center that specializes in lung disease.

Mr. Carraway, a patient of mine for the past two years, was admitted to the hospital for shortness of breath. He is a man with a long history of hypertension, kidney disease, and several past adverse reactions to prescription drugs. I was not working that weekend and neither was Dr. Hope, the doctor to whom Mr. Carraway was incorrectly assigned. The doctor covering for Dr. Hope assumed that Mr. Carraway had been seen by Dr. Hope in the past, even though Mr. Carraway told him he had not been. Thus Dr. Hope's cover ordered heart studies that were unnecessary and of course billed for a doctor's visit Mr. Carraway should never have had. The next day, only after Mr. Carraway insisted that I was his physician, I was called to see him, too late to stop the echocardiogram that was done for no reason or to prevent a worthless visit by an internist whose only participation in the patient's care was the bill he sent to the patient's insurance company.

Mr. Jay is an elderly man with what we call end-stage heart disease. He was admitted with severe heart failure and perhaps thirty pounds of extra water in his lungs, abdomen, and legs. It is important in such cases for the patient to keep his legs elevated, but after two days of requests we were unable to get him a stool to keep his legs up when he sat in a chair. After I told the head nurse I was going to write in the chart that we couldn't get a stool for the patient, a stool was found. Daily weights were ordered, but were not done for two days. Daily weights and measurement of urine output are ways of determining if we are effectively removing the excess fluid that accumulates in patients with heart failure. If we cannot get these precise measurements, we cannot be sure if the therapy is working. Strict measurements of his urine output were ordered, but they were deemed inaccurate, a very common occurrence in most hospitals where I've worked. Many physicians are so desperate to get an accurate account of how much urine their patient produces in a day that they will have the nurses place a Foley catheter in the patient's bladder. Then the urine volume can be easily measured, since it flows into a large bag with measurements on the side. But as I told you earlier in the chapter, these catheters can also lead to life-threatening urinary infections.

Mr. D is an elderly gentleman who had undergone coronary artery bypass surgery (CABG) that week. Three days after his operation, his family called to tell me that the surgical team told them he would be going to a rehab center the next day. They were quite upset that such an old man would be sent home so soon and also questioned me about why he was being sent to such a small rehab center: a four-bed room in a small hospital. First, I told the family that Mr. D would not be kicked out of the hospital the next day and that if he were to go to a rehab center, he would be sent to a center of excellence, not a four-bed room in a hospital that had some sort of relationship with our hospital.

Two days later, while still in the hospital and still on a monitor (thank God), Mr. D developed an irregular rhythm. Because he was without symptoms, my bet is that had he been sent to the rehab center, no one would have noticed. Instead, we were able to treat him with blood thinners and thus prevent him from having a stroke.

These stories, all of which are true, occurred during the course of only one week. The scary part is that I am sure that many doctors at almost any other hospital could write a similar narrative.

A Patient's Right to Dignity

I think it is important to add here that it is imperative not only that you survive your hospital stay but that your time in the hospital, which after all can last for days, weeks, months, or more, should not rob you of your dignity and self-respect in spite of what can often be rather humbling circumstances.

The loss of one's dignity is perhaps almost as damaging to a human being as the loss of one's health. If you have diarrhea and you need help to go to the bathroom ten times a day, well, then someone should be there for you at a moment's notice ten times a day. In reality, as we all know, many people end up soiling themselves and their bed. I've seen untouched meals taken away by orderlies because no one bothered to wake up a sleeping patient. I've seen many of my patients go thirsty because their pitcher of water is left out of their reach or because they are too frail to pour it. The elderly and the infirm who nevertheless have all their faculties frequently arrive at the hospital and soon find that their dignity is in as great a danger as their health. And it is perfectly obvious to me that a person's health suffers in direct relation to the diminishment of his or her dignity.

Years ago, like any other naïve third-year medical student, I walked the wards of the city hospitals. I can still remember on my first day hearing elderly patients crying out in vain for water or a bedpan. At first, with only the best of intentions, I either gave them a hand or found the nurse who was supposed to be caring for them. Some nurses, I am ashamed to say, in what I can only describe as a grotesque form of lassitude or entitlement, found my request to be an affront, as if asking them to do their job was nothing short of scandalous. Others, however, did help, and without complaint. God bless these compassionate souls, wherever they are found.

Within a month of my introduction to the ward, though, I cannot deny that I developed a certain all-too-common callousness when confronted with this same sort of situation. I was of course very busy, but I would often walk past a dimly lit room, no matter how plaintive the cry for help from within. Sometimes I would ask the nurse to do something, but other times, if I was exhausted or too busy or frankly just plain intimidated by the glares from the nurses' station, I just kept going on with my own work and on to my own patients.

I'm not sure if the situation was ever any better in hospitals, even decades ago. They had large, open wards where sometimes twenty or more men and women shared the same room, breathed the same air, heard the same croaking pleas for assistance, and passed back and forth the same infections. Hospitals today are surely better equipped in many ways. For the most part, the rooms are private, or at least semiprivate. (Some older hospitals, however, still have rooms with four beds in them, and I would urge you never to allow yourself to be admitted to a room like that.) The beds are better, the rooms have better air circulation and better lighting, and there are televisions at your bedside (although that will cost you at least $5 a day).

But there is also a terrible amount of apathy to be found within even the finest hospitals, and I all too frequently find that my patients' complaints are not about their illnesses but about the nurses' bell they have to ring over and over again in an attempt to get help.

There are no guaranteed solutions to this problem. I've already mentioned in this chapter the practical necessity of hiring someone to watch over you or your loved one, especially after leaving intensive care and returning to the regular floor, and suggested that if you cannot afford to purchase help, you should make every effort to have family members stay by your bedside. And my number one rule is *never* put up with abuse from the staff. If that sort of treatment occurs, I recommend that you consider having yourself moved to another hospital, even if you are pleased with your doctor.

Finally, it is the nature of our society itself, and not just the hospitals and the unions, which sets the tone of patient care, and thus it is up to us as a civilized society to step up and try to fix this problem. Nursing and ancillary staff numbers should be increased dramatically, and those whose skills or bedside manner are found seriously lacking or who are unsympathetic or apathetic and just plain burned out should be fired (instead of being given thirty or more warnings and meetings with a union rep). More of the young and the elderly should be encouraged to volunteer to aid in patient care. I am proud to say that as a sixteen-year-old I made beds, filled pitchers of water, and fed the elderly as a volunteer in a city hospital. I think my volunteer work gave me an incentive to study hard and an impetus to learn more about medicine. And I know for a fact that many of the healthy elderly, who are frequently lonely, often find new friends and a worthy way to spend their time as volunteers.

I hope you have developed a better understanding of the entire issue of hospitalization and perhaps also more than a little fear about the care you or someone dear to you might receive in any one of the thousands of hospitals across the country. Do your homework, get the best hospital, and once you are there, insist on receiving the best possible care. If we all did this we might put a few hospitals or doctors out of business.

In summary, here are my recommendations on how to survive your hospital stay:

1. An ounce of prevention is worth a pound of cure. Stay in shape, don't smoke, drive with caution, see a good doctor, and you'll be less likely to end up in a hospital.
2. In an emergency, go to a university hospital. Confront the ambulance driver if he tells you he is unable to take you to the hospital of your choice. This is especially true if you think you are having a heart attack.
3. Always carry with you a list of medications, allergies, and diagnoses and the name and telephone number of your doctor.
4. Make sure the emergency-room doctor calls your physician.
5. Consider transferring out of the hospital if you feel your treatment is poor.

6. Always question why a test is being done on you.

7. Write down your blood pressure and vital signs when they are done and if they seem incorrect or don't make sense, ask your doctor to double-check them.

8. Keep a record of the medications you are receiving and make sure you get the right ones. This is especially true in an emergency room, where the staff can forget to give you your usual daily medications.

9. Do not volunteer for any studies. Doctors make money and you take the risk.

10. Have a family member with you if you are being transported for special studies. In fact, have family members with you as much as possible; you may not have the strength to request things that you need. Bells ring for a long time in hospitals.

11. If you are in the hospital for an extended stay, ask a family member to call you before you go to bed to ask how you feel: How is your breathing, do you have any discomfort anywhere in your body, etc.

12. If you have a noisy roommate, get a new room. Call the administrator's office if you have to and threaten to report him or her if you do not have a clean and quiet room.

13. Don't let the hospital transfer you out of the intensive care unit or discharge you from the hospital if you think you are not ready. Call your doctor or even the hospital administrator if you are not satisfied.

Tricks of the Trade— How Some Doctors Are Taking Advantage of You and the System

Most physicians devote their lives to the practice of medicine in order to help others and, as the maxim goes, "First, do no harm." Yet, there are doctors who for whatever reason— basic human greed, overreaching ambition, flamboyant lifestyle, bad or illegal habits, spendthrift spouse—go out of their way to create additional revenue streams at the expense of the patient and his or her insurance company. In this chapter I'd like to tell you about several medical specialties, just as examples, and illustrate some of the unscrupulous ways in which some physicians deviate from their Hippocratic oath in pursuit of wealth.

The Primary-Care Physician

The primary-care physician, also called an internist or general doctor, serves as the principal conduit between the patient and all the other specialty physicians. He or she decides, essentially, when and where the patient should go for lab tests, for imaging exams, and for any and all other specialists' opinions. Your primary-care physician should be the doctor you know the best and the one you trust the most. There are countless PCPs who combine great skill, humanity, and dedication to their work, and in a previous chapter I have given my suggestions on how best to find a highly qualified primary-care physician.

Compared to the specialist, however, the primary-care doctor often has fewer years of training, and it is more likely that he or she earns significantly less income. This great disparity in annual income—sometimes the difference between the annual million-dollar salary of a busy orthopedist and the low six-figure salary of an equally hardworking and dedicated internist—does create resentment and jealousy among some. In my twelve years of experience as a community physician, I have observed how frequently some doctors, even those who started out with the best intentions, end up engaged in a cutthroat competition.

For example, an internist or primary-care physician may reach a point in his career where he asks himself, "Why can't I perform these more elaborate tests myself?" A physician may charge as much as $600 for a sonogram of the heart, while he might charge as little as $40 for a patient visit. And yet it takes no more time to do a sonogram (which is in fact done by a technician) than it does for a doctor to see a patient. Simple math tells you that a doctor would have to see no fewer than fifteen patients to earn the same money he would bring in by doing one sonogram. If he did fifteen sonograms in the time it would take him to do fifteen patient visits, he could earn $9,000 instead of $600. Which method of producing income is more enticing?

Of course, it is morally corrupt and professionally reprehensible for an untrained physician to perform and interpret a sophisticated test. Cardiologists train an additional two to four years before they are comfortable in the use and interpretation of an echocardiogram (pictures of the heart that are taken in much the same way as those of a fetus on a sonogram and are then placed on a videotape and viewed on a VCR). However, in recent years a vastly greater number of medical doctors have somehow contrived a way to perform these studies. This is how they do it.

Most HMOs (health maintenance organizations) allow only cardiologists or radiologists to perform these exams, yet the biggest insurers in the country—Medicare and Medicaid—allow any physician to do them. Thus, many doctors purchase or lease a sonogram machine and perform all sorts of sonography (echo, carotid duplex, venous and arterial exams, abdominal exams) on their elderly patients and get paid handsomely for it. Some have their technicians read it for them and then just sign off on the results themselves. Others make deals with radiologists and cardiologists willing to read the studies at a bargain rate.

Over the past decade I have been asked countless times to read studies like these by physicians who administer the tests but are not equipped and trained to read the results. I have always declined, since most of these arrangements are scams created by doctors who haven't the slightest idea of how an echo machine works, what symptoms indicate the necessity for the study (save to get paid for it), or if their technician (the trained professional doing the study) is qualified to perform the study. Yet many less than scrupulous cardiologists do read the studies taken by untrained doctors, happy to pocket the small fees offered by their even less scrupulous colleagues. After all, reading ten studies one night at home on your VCR can bring you $400 to $500 (the medical doctor of course makes ten times that amount), and, more important, by getting into bed with the medical doctor, this cardiologist has formed a new relationship. Thus a new referral pattern begins. The honest cardiologist loses his patients and test referrals to this dishonest one, who proceeds to enrich himself in a shady manner and create a new referral base.

Should I have been amazed recently when it came to my attention that a fresh graduate of a cardiology program became one of the busiest cardiologists at several of the local hospitals? Not when I learned that he was employing schemes like the one described above. To make matters worse, the "if I don't do it, he will" scenario has taken medicine by storm. Rather than report their associates to the appropriate authorities, many physicians have become part of the same game, discarding their own ethics in order to double and triple and quadruple their profits.

The Hand-Off

Let's say a patient is transferred to another hospital for a special test, in this instance, for example, a cardiac angiogram. Logic dictates that the patient should be transferred to the service of the doctor who will be performing the procedure. What happens in some hospitals, however, is just a scheme to double- or even triple-bill. I call it the hand-off.

Instead of being admitted to that doctor's service, the patient finds himself under the care of an internist whom he has never even met. He in turn calls for a consultant. The consultant is the person who will be performing the important exams, the very individual who should have admitted the patient to begin with. Some of the more prestigious hospitals in New York City have been doing this for decades. Thus, every day the patient is seen by two doctors, and the patient or his or her insurance company gets billed by two physicians. It's a deal that the hospital may arrange or one the cardiology team might concoct. The internist is happy, since he collects perhaps $1,000 for unnecessary visits, and the cardiologist is happy because the internist (often a physician who refers patients to him) is happy. And because the responsibility for the small amount of paperwork that might need to be done is shared by his partner in crime.

In reality, all cardiologists have been trained in internal medicine and therefore should be able to care for a patient admitted for a cardiac procedure, even if the patient has some other general medical problems (diabetes, for example).

Perhaps the greatest abuse of this hand-off scheme concerns the weakest and most unfortunate part of our population: the elderly housed in nursing homes. Every day thousands of demented patients are sent from nursing homes to the local hospital. Physicians caring for these patients, in my opinion, are sometimes of dubious quality and possess less than sterling ethics. In order to make their visit with this unknowing and perhaps unwilling demented patient as limited as possible (although they bill for an extended visit), they call in several consultants. In other words, they hand off the responsibility of caring for the patient to others.

Let me give you a typical example. A ninety-two-year-old woman suffering from dementia is admitted to the hospital for shortness of breath. She is nonverbal, gets fed through a tube at the nursing home, and is not oriented. The "nursing-home doctor" admits the patient and calls in a pulmonologist (perhaps she has pneumonia), a cardiologist (perhaps she has heart failure), and a gastroenterologist (she is also slightly anemic). All of the work involved, i.e., checking the X ray, reviewing the data, and perhaps discussing the care and prognosis with the family, can and should be done by the nursing-home doctor, but instead he spends five minutes on the case and calls his friends in to figure it all out, and so they can each send their bill to Medicare. What should have been no more than a simple one-day visit for mild heart failure is thus turned into a weeklong visit of frightening and probing and billing for this ill-fated soul.

The Hospital-Employed Physician, a.k.a. the Full-Time Physician

I was astonished to learn that many physicians employed by hospitals are made to follow an unwritten rule: Always use the physicians or services available within a given hospital. Or, in other words, always support the hospital and not the physicians or services that might be available outside the hospital, regardless of the quality of a particular physician or lab. I call this one of the tricks of the trade because it suggests that doctors are obliged to call upon their hospital colleagues' services even when the latter are less qualified than someone whose office is half a block away but who is not affiliated with the hospital. Or they may send you to a doctor who works for the hospital for a procedure even though there is a three-month wait for an appointment. This is in my view a travesty and a blight upon the integrity of hospitals everywhere this practice occurs. I've heard of and from many physicians who complain about the terrible service they and their patients receive from the full-time faculty at their hospital but who continue to do what is right for their department and their future at the expense of what is right for the patient. In my efforts to document this reprehensible practice (once again, as before, it is always about the money), I located two signed memos from one of the highest-ranking doctors at a hospital: the chief of medicine.

In 1984, the chairman of the department of cardiology at a New York City hospital wished to drum up business for the heart surgeons who worked there. In my opinion, at that time the most qualified heart surgeon at the hospital, although technically a member of the hospital staff, was not a "hospital-employed physician." Thus, many of the cases and the payments that go along with them were going to that surgeon rather than to the hospital's physicians. To underscore his contempt for such activity, on March 16, 1984, Dr. James Scheuer, the chairman of the department of cardiology, sent out the following memo to all the full-time cardiologists at the institution. His purpose is clear.

In view of the statistics I reviewed with you at the Cardiology Faculty meeting of March 15th, I would appreciate it if for uncomplicated surgical cases you would consider using Drs. Brodman, Robinson, and Frater.[1] In uncomplicated cases, there are clearly no significant differences in mortality statistics among the major surgeons at this institution.

On August 12, 1992, the same Dr. Scheuer (now having been promoted to chairman of the Department of Medicine) became upset about a patient who had been sent to one of the newer private angiographers at the hospital. To discourage this rebellious act from occurring again, he wrote another memo to a staff member and in this one concluded: "I cannot understand why a new, untried interventionist, just out of fellowship, would be chosen in preference." This "untried" angiographer actually had at least as much if not more formal training than the angiographers employed at the institution and remains a well-respected and qualified doctor in his field.

As you can see, even chief doctors at large university hospitals are not ashamed of urging the doctors who work for them to send at least the easy cases (your mom or your dad, perhaps?) to less-qualified doctors who work for the institution. The hospital rewarded him for his efforts by elevating him to chairman of medicine, a position he held for many years. When he retired, there were galas and other ceremonies held in this honor.

Every hospital has its strong points and its weak points, its great departments and departments that are staffed with less than the very best doctors. Yet even at the best university hospitals it's almost unheard of that a doctor would send you crosstown to his or her competitor. So if you are a heart patient at hospital A, which recently began a heart transplant program, you are probably going to be sent to an unproven transplant program (or even worse, to a doctor with a terrible transplant record) instead of to the hospital only a few miles away with a time-tested high-quality heart transplant program. By the way, I'm not just suggesting this *might* occur; it is happening right now.

In other cases, patients are told they may need to wait months for a stress test, sonogram, or even an CAT scan because the hospital-affiliated lab is overwhelmed with cases and the doctors working for the hospital will not send their patients to a private outside lab, even if the doctors and the lab are better equipped and the wait for the patient is only a few days. So if you need a stress test right away and your doctor tells you that the next appointment is in three months, make the smart choice. Go elsewhere for the test and go elsewhere for all your care, since your doctor is not looking out for you.

In cardiology, the echo department is often one of the biggest moneymakers for a hospital. So, in many hospitals, private doctors are not permitted to interpret and be paid for reading the studies. For the most part, huge university hospitals have very high-quality doctors reading these studies, but in the smaller hospitals it's almost a first-come/first-served principle. Older doctors, sometimes without much training, may have exclusivity in reading echoes even though they do a terrible job of it. Again, another reason to seek care at a quality teaching hospital.

No-Show Rent

How can a physician pay another to send him patients? I call this scam the phantom or no-show rent scenario. It is a way of making a kickback scheme (you send me patients and I'll give you cash) look like an honest transaction. The physician, Dr. A, usually a general practitioner or internist, rents space to a specialist, Dr. B, often at an above-market rate, and in return for his monthly "rent" check, A sends his patients to his new tenant, B. Often B never even shows up at the office. I'm not saying that doctors who pay fair market rate for office space are doing anything wrong here, but I am saying that the others, and they are the majority, are involved in a not-so-complex scam. I know of one cardiologist who, according to his rental agreements, had six different office locations. Of course he has no phone or desk at these locations, but if asked to produce some sort of rental contract, I suspect his lawyer could.

The Urologist—the Kidney Stone Caper

In small community hospitals and, yes, even in the parking lots of doctor's offices, a procedure called shock-wave lithotripsy is being performed in record numbers. At first glance, one might assume that there is an unexpectedly high incidence of kidney stones in certain areas of the country. Shock-wave lithotripsy is a noninvasive way of pulverizing stones that are in the urinary system into sandlike particles that can then be passed out in the urine. The procedure offers many benefits to both the patient and the insurance company. It is a relatively inexpensive, noninvasive, and safe procedure that does not require admission to the hospital or an operating room.

Imagine, however, that hundreds of these procedures are being performed on patients who don't even have kidney stones. I recently became aware of this "caper" thanks to some reputable and concerned urologists (kidney surgeons) and technicians who are on staff at a small community hospital. According to several sources, these inappropriate procedures have been going on in front of the hospital administrators' closed eyes for years.

The scam starts when a primary-care physician refers a patient to one of these unethical urologists. Some of these MDs giving referrals may be friends of these doctors, while others are just innocent physicians, unwitting participants in this scam. The patient may be referred because of symptoms like back pain, blood in the urine, or an infection in the urinary system. Another reason may be microscopic hematuria (blood in the urine only seen under the microscope). Kidney stones are one of many reasons a person might have blood in the urine.

It seems that a diagnostic evaluation is often then done by the less than reputable urologist in his office. This includes X rays and sonograms, and the results are often fabricated by a very simple sleight of hand in order to indicate the presence of a stone. In some cases, a patient with no stone is simply given the X ray of another patient who actually has or had one. In other cases, a phlebolith, a calcification of soft tissue that is not a stone, is purposely misread by the urologist as a stone to provide the necessary validation for performing what is in fact an unnecessary procedure. In still other cases, a patient with an actual stone undergoes the procedure, unaware that his trusted doctor purposefully leaves part of the stone in place so that the patient has to return for another round of shock-wave lithotripsy.

I have met with and spoken to other urologists who have been involved with these doctors or who have actually reviewed their records. They confirmed that patients they saw for a second opinion sometimes had no stones or did not have stones amenable to this technique. Unfortunately, no one has had the courage to come forward and expose this unconscionable and illegal behavior. I suspect that these doctors have rationalized this entire charade, justified it in some way that allows them to look themselves in the mirror every morning. After all, they are "doing no harm."

I can only assume that this hospital is but one of many harboring doctors who perform unnecessary shock-wave lithotripsy. I hope that those who read this section will think twice before they blindly trust their doctor's opinion on the subject of kidney stones. And at the very least, always get a second opinion.

The Kidney Doctor—the Nephrologist

Most of us will never need to see a kidney doctor, and thankfully only a small handful of us will need to be placed on dialysis for kidney failure, but it is here in the dialysis center that some unethical physicians are known to misbehave. At present I only know for sure of one group that seems to be doing this (years ago I was asked to participate in this madness but I declined), but I imagine there must be many more greedy nephrologists out there who are doing the same.

You're a special client when you are a patient of a dialysis center. Since your kidneys cannot remove the poisons from your blood, you are required to have them removed by a dialysis machine. A normal procedure lasts for several hours and occurs three days a week, every week of your life. Usually these centers have several machines running at once, and as a result several patients sit there, perhaps reading or watching television, until the process is completed. Unfortunately, some of the doctors who run these centers keep the patients occupied with other games, most notably tests. I'll explain.

First, they receive echocardiograms to rule out any new heart disease or perhaps the presence of some abnormal fluid that may have accumulated around the heart. Neither condition is uncommon in these patients, but nevertheless, neither should be sought unless there is some clinical reason to suspect that something is going on. Since most of the patients are insured by Medicare (our government does that to make sure these people get cared for) and since Medicare doesn't really check to see if these studies are necessary (described in Chapter 7, "Medicine in Crisis"), the doctors usually get paid around $450 per echocardiogram.

During my interviews with several nephrologists, I was told that some of the doctors are also finding ways to get more bang for their buck when administering the drug Epogen (Amgen Labs) to their dialysis patients. Epogen can reverse the anemia often seen in patients with kidney failure. It is also one of the very few drugs (see the section on oncologists, page 117) that a doctor can order and then sell to the patient's insurance company. It is sold in a vial to the doctor and usually given as an injection to the patient during his or her dialysis. It's truly a wonder drug. The manufacturer tops off (they call it "overfill") the vial with an extra 1,000 units of the drug for expected waste (some is lost in the syringe while clearing the needle, etc.). I've been told, however, that some of the doctors are finding ways of saving the extra 1,000 units and combining enough of them— usually five—to come up with another dose. Thus, for every five patients they get a free dose and bill Medicare a full charge.

I think this practice is illegal. It certainly increases the risk of contamination of the product, which is injected into the patient, since as I mentioned, you have to take small (one hopes sterile) quantities from several different vials until you have enough for an extra dose. If any of those in Medicare were paying attention they could contact the pharmaceutical supply house, do some simple math, and then levy huge fines on these doctors and stop this unethical, penny-pinching process.

The Gastroenterologist

The gastroenterologist earns a significant percentage of his or her income through the administration of a test called an endoscopy. This procedure is performed by placing a tiny camera into the stomach or rectum so as to give those areas a complete visual inspection. It is without doubt one of the most important exams for any patient with symptoms of, or who is at risk for, cancer. Asymptomatic patients over the age of fifty, and patients with a strong family history of cancer once they reach the age of forty, are strongly urged to have a colonoscopy. A doctor can easily remove a precancerous growth (called a polyp), and in so doing he can essentially remove the risk of that growth becoming frank colon cancer.

Despite the obvious importance of the procedure, many physicians are using it far too often simply to create additional income. Physicians not certified in the procedure are performing it in the office (it is harder for noncertified physicians to get such privileges at a hospital). Since perforation of the intestine, the major risk in having a colonoscopy, is quite low (2 in 1,000), it is unusual for untrained physicians to cause harm.

The greatest abuse, however, takes place when a physician removes a polyp. In that instance, he is able to bill for a separate procedure and can increase his fee by almost 50 percent. In addition, if the physician finds a polyp, he has an excuse to perform another exam within a few years to look for more polyps. While most physicians I know remove only true polyps, it is well known that there are other doctors who perform removal of what are called "suction-induced polyps."

A suction-induced polyp is a polyp created by the doctor at the time of the procedure. Essentially, he places a suction catheter against the wall of the intestine and sucks a small piece up until it looks like a polyp. Then the doctor photographs the polyp for documentation and takes a biopsy of it. The risk of perforation of the intestine wall is also increased by this sort of bogus biopsy.

The Cancer Doctors—
the Oncologist and the Surgeon

As a third-year medical student, my first rotation in a doctor's office was with an oncologist, a physician specializing in the treatment of cancer. My first memory from the first hour of my first day there is of sitting in his office and watching while the physician scolded his nurse for not charging the patient he had just seen more money for his services. The patient had a deadly form of cancer known as multiple myeloma. Since then I have met some very compassionate and wonderful oncologists, but I have met some others who are without a doubt the most treacherous people in the medical field.

Oncologists are given a special privilege: They can not only order drugs, specifically chemotherapy drugs, but they can also dispense and bill for them. No other doctor can do this. This entices some of these reprehensible, cynical, and greedy individuals to administer chemotherapy to patients indiscriminately in spite of its horrible, potentially lethal adverse effects and very unlikely benefits. They purchase drug A and can bill a significant multiple of their cost to you or your insurance company. The more chemo they give, the more money they make. It is for this reason that any patients diagnosed with a form of malignant cancer must seek at least a second or even a third opinion.

Positive-sounding medical jargon like *positive response, shrinkage,* or *partial remission* very often means nothing in terms of the patient's overall mortality. Surgeons often tell the patient's family that they were able to remove *most* of the cancer. With cancer, however, if you don't remove the entire tumor and afterward annihilate any of the microscopic cells still remaining, you will not survive. So why let Grandma receive poisonous and devastating chemotherapy if the oncologist cannot show you published data that support giving it to her? Or why go through lung surgery if another surgeon tells you the tumor is inoperable? Why does our society allow doctors affiliated with nursing homes to administer chemotherapy to demented and terminal patients or even to perform pointless surgery on them?

The Cardiac Catheterization—Heart Angiogram

The cardiac catheterization, also known as a heart angiogram, is usually performed by specialists trained in the field of cardiology and with further training (we hope) in the subspecialty of heart angiograms. They are often referred to as angiographers. At a recent meeting of angiographers, the members were asked three questions. They were asked to raise their hand if they thought some of their colleagues performed nonindicated (unnecessary) cardiac angiograms on patients. Almost all those present raised their hands. They were then asked if they knew someone in that room who performed nonindicated cardiac angiograms. Again, almost everyone raised his hand. Finally, they were asked if they ever performed nonindicated cardiac catheterizations. This time, not surprisingly, no one raised his hand.

Cardiac catheterizations are currently performed in hospitals with and without cardiac surgical backup.[2] According to the Society for Cardiac Angiography and Interventions, there are more than 2,100 cardiac catheterization laboratories in the United States (including Puerto Rico and the Virgin Islands). Of these labs, 72 percent provided on-site cardiac surgery (which means that 28 percent of the hospitals could not provide bypass surgery). Fifty-eight laboratories were located in nonhospital settings (doctor's offices, parking lots, etc.). It is estimated that almost 2 million cardiac catheterizations were performed in this country in 1993 and that by 2010, the number will be up to 3 million yearly.[3] In addition, according to the American Heart Association, 561,000 percutaneous transluminal coronary angioplasties (PTCAs), with or without stents, were performed.[4] Based on the responses to the questions in the meeting, the reader can understand that not all of these risky and expensive procedures are necessary. Although the American College of Cardiology publishes guidelines for the indications of coronary angiograms (*www.acc.org*), there are equivocal indications that give some physicians, in their own minds, anyway, enough justification to perform the study. In almost every hospital in this country, there are physicians performing nonindicated studies and placing metallic stents in the arteries of patients unnecessarily. It has been estimated that in many of these centers as many as 15 to 18 percent of these angiograms are done for "inappropriate indications."[5] Qualified doctors often stand around in amazement as unqualified or greedy doctors wheel unfortunate and misinformed patients into the lab to undergo unnecessary procedures.

Most frequently, the patient is told that there was a blockage of an important artery and that it was opened by the procedure.

While this may be true, studies show that many of these patients will have no significant benefit (reduction in mortality or symptoms) from the procedure. Thus, billions of health-care dollars are being thrown away.

The Plastic Surgeon

I've already written about my feelings concerning physicians who put glitzy ads in local newspapers. Not very professional, is it? But for plastic surgeons in particular, this tawdry way of getting business is endemic. Open up an issue of *New York* magazine, for example, and you'll see plenty different plastic surgeons yearning to do a tummy tuck, liposuction, or face-lift. At about $4,000 for an eighth-of-a-page ad that runs for months at a time, these doctors are spending lots of money on marketing and promotion that they need to recoup.

Physicians who perform cosmetic surgery seem to be multiplying faster than bunny rabbits. That's because board-certified plastic surgeons are not the only ones performing this type of surgery. So are dermatologists (especially facial peels and hair transplants to make you look younger). And urologists. Would you believe radiologists?! As sick as this may sound, some of the doctors out there giving Botox injections and performing hair transplants took a quickie course and now are advertising themselves as experts in the field. I would be willing to bet that many of these doctors left their previous profession because they weren't very good at it. Or maybe they just wanted to make some easy money.

And for those patients who assume that just about any doctor can administer the drug, even Allergan, the manufacturer of Botox, places the following statement in their prescribing information to physicians: "Physicians administering BOTOX COSMETIC must understand the relevant neuromuscular and/or orbital anatomy of the area involved and any alterations to the anatomy due to prior surgical procedures." The manufacturer's FDA-approved and required statement is there because there is a risk of causing too much weakness of a muscle with an improper dosage. If, for example, the muscle in the eyelid is weakened to such an extent that you cannot close your eye, you run the risk of damaging your cornea. Trust me, most physicians, including this author, have no understanding of the complex anatomy of the eye, so please find yourself a board-certified and experienced cosmetic surgeon, and not some unemployed or moonlighting urologist or radiologist, if you wish to remove some age lines by using Botox.

I have urged you to find the best primary-care doctor possible. If you have chosen wisely and you feel you must have some form of cosmetic surgery, your PCP is the one who can help you find a good plastic surgeon and not some shyster advertising in a magazine.

I have spoken with plastic surgeons on many occasions. Even interviewed some. As a fellow physician, I confess I have long been suspicious of all the different ways the greedy and unscrupulous types among them prey upon mankind's eternal obsession with physical appearance. Some will perform bizarre types of surgery, including buttock implants for women and chest implants for men. I've even been told of surgeons doing implants to lengthen feet. Are we so vain that we must worry about the length of our feet? And are these surgeries recognized as effective and safe?

Perhaps the most abused procedure of all is liposuction. Qualified and honest surgeons tell me that they will turn away men and women who are morbidly obese rather than lie to them about the benefits of liposuction. I am told that if you are morbidly obese to begin with, even the most aggressive liposuction will have only limited results. But others in the field surely are not so scrupulous.

And then there are the payment scams, seen only in the medical world for service in the field of cosmetic surgery. You may have noticed that many doctors, in order to attract more (gullible) customers, promote a monthly payment plan in their advertisements for those who cannot afford to cough up the entire fee at the time of the procedure. You know the drill; it is as if you are buying something on QVC. You want to have some liposuction done, but the procedure costs a whopping $4,000! No problem, says the kindhearted doctor. You only need to pay a finance company $200 a month. For forty months! The surgeon gets paid $3,500 up front by the finance company for a procedure he normally would charge $4,000 for, and you end up paying $8,000 in installments.

The Little Things All Add Up

Everyone has had the following experience. You go to the store to purchase a vacuum cleaner that's on sale for $100, but before you can get back out the door, the salesperson has talked you into buying a fancier hose and a power vac, extra belts, carpet cleaner, special filter bags, and a two-year warranty. Your total cost now is well over $200.

Imagine for a moment that your trusted primary-care physician might also be a very good and very motivated salesperson. Remember also that you are conditioned not to be on guard against any kind of hard sell since, after all, your insurance company is going to pay for everything or almost everything anyway.

An initial visit with a primary-care physician is usually billed at about $125. It consists of a comprehensive history and a physical exam, which can take about thirty minutes to an hour, or so the code books suggest. However, if one were to add a chest X ray, EKG, urine analysis, blood tests, spirometry, an abdominal sonogram, and a flexible sigmoidoscopy, the bill might be nearly $1,000. You can see how the little things start to really add up.

When I ask patients whether this is a common experience, they almost unanimously agree. Moreover, I find that most people appear to prefer it when they have these tests done by their physician and in that physician's office. After all, it doesn't cost patients anything, it is more convenient, and they leave feeling that they have been thoroughly checked out. However, the reality is that many of these tests are unnecessary or, at the very least, should not be performed by a primary-care physician.

Chest X Ray

There are several reputable studies that tell us that yearly chest X rays do nothing to increase the chance of survival if a cancer is found. In fact, most policies state that a chest X ray is not recommended as part of a periodic medical examination unless justified by symptoms, signs, or change in status of a chronic condition. Yet how many of you continue to get yearly routine chest X rays? In addition, most physicians, other than radiologists, do not have enough training or knowledge to be considered reliable interpreters of these studies. Therefore, I urge you to at least ask your physician why he or she is recommending this study and if the American College of Physicians (ACP) suggests having the study done. Alas, my fear is that many will not even know. If you both agree that there are compelling reasons why a chest X ray should be performed, I would insist that your doctor send you to a facility where board-certified radiologists and their trained staff will perform and interpret your exam. Finally, I would advise you to request that a copy of the report be sent to your home.

Spirometry (Lung Test)

This is the all-too-familiar exam where the patient blows into a small machine. The simple, straightforward type of spirometry can be performed by an internist, but the more sophisticated spirometry, which involves a study of lung diffusion, should be performed only by a board-certified pulmonologist. In general, patients who are not suffering from significant shortness of breath, prolonged cough, or wheezing should not have this test. Thus, in my opinion, the vast majority of physicians who routinely perform this procedure on their new patients are just doing it to pad the bill and increase their income.

The Blood Test

We should all have a blood test on an initial exam. A fasting cholesterol test should probably be done on everyone when he or she reaches the age of twenty. A select few should have it done in their teens. These blood tests can be run on small analyzers in the physician's office, by large industrial machines in the hospital, or at an independent lab. Your physician will benefit financially from such tests if he has his own lab facilities. If he sends your sample to an independent lab or hospital, you can assume that his motives are unimpeachable and purely altruistic. From a quality-control perspective, it is also worth noting that the industrial machines are monitored and maintained by a full-time lab technician, whereas the unit in the doctor's office might instead be serviced by the receptionist in the doctor's office. Thus, when you need blood tests, make sure the blood is sent to an independent lab that accepts your insurance.

Sigmoidoscopy—Screening for Colon Cancer

The Balanced Budget Act of 1997 provided all Medicare beneficiaries coverage for a screening sigmoidoscopy and fecal-occult-blood testing. The American Cancer Society and the American Gastroenterological Association recommend periodic flexible sigmoidoscopies in all patients over the age of fifty but only recommend a complete colonoscopy for those patients considered at high risk for colon cancer.[6]

An internist or gastroenterologist performs a flexible sigmoidoscopy, although, quite frankly, few internists or general doctors have any significant training in this procedure. It employs a flexible hose with a small video camera at the end that can see only about twenty centimeters into the rectum and colon. A colonoscopy is a much longer version of the scope and can be advanced through the entire colon. The colonoscopy enables the practitioner not only to look for signs of a growth in the colon but also to biopsy the lesion and often remove it altogether. This procedure should be performed *only* by a board-certified gastroenterologist. I stress the word *only* because many general doctors are presently performing this procedure.

Two recent studies published in the July 20, 2000, *New England Journal of Medicine* concluded that a significant number of cancerous lesions were missed when patients were screened with a sigmoidoscope instead of a colonoscope because they were out of the range of the sigmoidoscope. Physicians therefore strongly suggest that patients without risk factors have a full colonoscopy when they reach the age of fifty, and that high-risk patients have the study much sooner, perhaps as early as age forty.[7]

Thus, if your physician wishes to perform a flexible sigmoidoscopy, I suggest you request that he or she send you to a board-certified gastroenterologist for a full screening colonoscopy. As per my pervious suggestions, always get the name of at least two different specialists, weigh your options, and make an educated decision from there.

ECG—Electrocardiogram

The ECG (also called EKG) is a simple procedure performed by placing ten electrodes on the patient's body. I am sure most of you have had one. Essentially, it records the electrical output of the heart in twelve different directions. It is a simple test that can detect ongoing or old heart attacks, abnormal rhythms of the heart, or abnormalities in the conduction throughout the heart. A good computerized interpretation is accurate over 90 percent of the time (probably more accurate than the average physician). An ECG can also double the cost of a routine visit (about $45).

The American College of Cardiology and the American Heart Association published guidelines in 1992 describing all the situations in which electrocardiograms are useful. First and foremost, everyone forty years and older should have a baseline ECG (previous AHA guidelines suggested an ECG be done at age twenty). In my personal opinion, any patient twenty years and older should have an ECG when seeing a doctor for the first time. It goes without saying that a baseline ECG is considered appropriate for all patients with either suspected cardiovascular conditions or those at high risk for developing such conditions. It is also considered an appropriate test after administration of any drug known to influence cardiac conduction. It is not recommended that patients who have remained clinically stable have follow-up electrocardiograms more than once a year, unless they have been previously demonstrated to have cardiac disease. Electrocardiograms are considered appropriate before all types of surgery in patients in this group.[8]

I am quite certain that many of you reading this book are thirty years old and quite healthy and are getting an ECG every time you see your physician. If your condition is stable and you've been given an ECG more than once a year, you and your insurance company may have been abused.

Sonography—Echocardiogram, Carotid Duplex, Abdominal Sonogram, Arterial and Venous Doppler

Most of you know what a sonogram is. It is a machine that can image certain organs or vascular structures through the use of sound waves. Whether imaging your baby-to-be, your heart, your liver, etc., the machine is essentially the same for each. However, the interpretation of these different structures requires a separate expertise. A cardiologist might be an expert at looking at the heart, but he or she wouldn't know much about imaging a uterus, and so on.

So, if your general doctor is performing any of these tests in his office, I would suggest you find another doctor immediately. Your doctor has no legitimate training in doing these studies, interpreting them, or even establishing when or why to order them. It is nothing more or less than an improper and potentially dangerous way for the physician to generate a bill for $1,000 or more out of a visit that should only cost $50. I have called the fraud hotline numbers of three large insurance carriers to register complaints about such instances as this, and to my astonishment, I have yet to receive a response from them. Perhaps this inattention and fiscal irresponsibility are the reasons why the great majority of HMOs have consistently failed to be profitable in recent years.

If your doctor thinks you should have one of these tests, I would suggest you ask him to send you to a board-certified physician or to a teaching hospital to have it done. If he tells you that the studies are done in his office but are read by a radiologist or cardiologist, I would be very suspicious that he has some scheme arranged with the doctor who is reading them. Again, go somewhere else.

I must admit that about ten years ago when my partner and I first began practicing cardiology, we saw an opportunity to perform echoes in nursing homes and at some physician's offices. At the time, we thought we could market the idea as a great convenience for their patients, but we were quite naïve in our dealings with other doctors. We hired a law firm that specialized in medical legal issues and followed their suggestions. In many cases we went to offices of very honorable doctors with a signed lease agreement based upon a customary fee for the use of the office and their secretarial staff, usually no more than $250 to $500/month. While this worked out for all initially (patients were happy that they did not need to travel, and we improved our business), some of the doctors began to demand more and more money and new leases from us.

After a year or so we had to abandon our plan because of these greedy and unethical requests. As I said, we were naïve to the world of medicine, and I regret we ever even tried to do it. Since that time, as you will see, all sorts of echo arrangements are being made in medicine. But I can say unequivocally that it is best to get an echo (if you truly need one) at a board-certified cardiologist's office with the cardiologist present, in case the technician has a question for him or her at the time of the study. So even if Mom or Dad is in a rehab facility or nursing home (unless they are too ill to travel), have them sent to the cardiologist's office for the study instead of having a technician come to them.

I would venture a guess that at present at least 20 percent of the general doctors in the New York area are involved in echo schemes. Many of them hire a technician, lease an echo machine, and perform echoes on everyone they can. Some doctors just let the technician read the study, and to make it look legit they sign the report themselves. Others pay a cardiologist a small fee to read the study. As part of this deal, however, the family doctor may call this cardiologist (rather than those who refuse to play in the scheme) for all his consultations. Those cardiologists who refuse to help interpret these studies are penalized by the family doctors; they don't get consults anymore.

I'm sure that thousands of you have been sold the same bill of goods (or in this case, an echo) by your family doctor. I would also guess that as many as a million echoes are done every year for no good reason. Based on the cost of nearly $500 per test, it is costing the insurance companies $500 million to pay for them. Ever wonder why you pay so much for your health insurance?

As a cardiologist, I have been trained to interpret echocardiograms. However, many cardiologists with my level of training or less are also performing and interpreting carotid duplex studies, which look at the arteries in the neck, and venous and arterial studies of the legs, since they pay very well. I am willing to bet that most of them have never had formal training in these more arcane procedures. I refuse to do these studies even though the machine I have can perform them. I would urge any patient to see only a competent board-certified vascular surgeon, preferably in a large teaching hospital, for these studies.

The Exercise Stress Test

A general doctor, in my opinion, should almost never perform an exercise stress test. While there may be exceptions, only a cardiologist has received adequate training to perform this test properly. If you are interested in the indication for or the appropriateness of exercise testing, you can review this in most cardiology textbooks, like Braunwald's *A Textbook in Cardiology*, online at *www.acc.org*, or in the source cited in the notes section.[9]

Most readers might say that there can be little harm in having a stress test. Indeed, the physical risk involved in having a stress test is quite insignificant. However, if the study is misinterpreted as abnormal or if the test is read as falsely positive (the test is abnormal, but your heart is normal), you may then be forced to have a more complicated stress test, called a nuclear stress test.

Let's say you are a thirty-eight-year-old woman with mild hypertension but no other risk factors for heart disease and your doctor sends you for a stress test because once in a while you get a fleeting, sharp, stabbing pain in your chest that lasts one or two seconds. I just consulted on a patient who came to me with this history and an abnormal stress test as well as an abnormal nuclear stress test. In a patient like Mrs. C (who has a very low likelihood of having coronary artery disease) the chance of that abnormal regular stress test being incorrectly abnormal (falsely positive) is very likely. Even a more advanced study, which involved an injection of a nuclear agent into her body to image her heart (also noted as mildly abnormal), is also more often incorrectly abnormal. It's just a game of statistics known to the experts as Bayesian analysis of stress tests, and it is the reason why good doctors don't perform procedures on patients with a very low likelihood of having a truly abnormal result.

The patient and I were now faced with either ignoring the test she should have never had in the first place, worrying about her imminent demise, or having her undergo an angiogram, which can cause stroke, heart attack, or death (even in the best of hands) in about 3 out of 1,000 cases. All because her doctor was unfamiliar with published guidelines for conducting stress tests (*www.acc.org*) or perhaps because the doctor was interested in making a few extra dollars. The patient might have figured that since the test wouldn't cost her anything (her insurance would pick up the expense), there was no risk. No test or medicine is without risk, even if it is free!

By the way, I chose to tell her never to go back to her doctor, to lose weight, and begin an exercise program.

Should Your Doctor's Office Be a Store?

It probably will not surprise you to learn that I am very suspicious of physicians who sell products from their office. Oncologists are permitted to sell drugs (in this case, chemotherapy) directly to the patient or the insurance company. With few exceptions, however, most medical practitioners cannot sell drugs and thus don't have yet another incentive to prescribe costly medications to you. So what can a doctor sell you in his office?

Vitamins, skin products, and weight-control formulas are the most common things. Since these are not prescription drugs, doctors are permitted to sell you their magic potions. Often, you pay double or triple the price for a simple vitamin manufactured in a huge lab that caters to the physician. Labels like "Doctor So-and-So's Health Vitamin" are produced by the company and slapped on bottles of vitamins that are shipped to the doctor. And that's not all. Not only are these supplements sold to you without any scientific proof of their effectiveness or safety, they may not even contain what the label says they do. That's because there are no FDA requirements for these manufacturers, whether these products are sold in your doctor's office, health food stores, or on television.

The companies that sell these products to your physician don't just drop the product off, either. They also supply marketing schemes, signs, and false scientific statements. Some even provide special payment plans for the doctor's patients.

Perhaps the biggest culprits in these schemes are the dermatologists. During your appointment, the physician or his nurse extols the virtues of products that he claims he has developed or sells exclusively for a company. It's hard to refuse to purchase a product from the person who is treating you and who tells you that this product will make you better. Your skin is blemished, maybe you are dating someone, and you are going to disagree with the doctor who wants to help you? So what's another $200 if it will make you look better? But what if these products could be purchased for a fraction of the cost at the local pharmacy? Or what if a better alternative medication is covered under your insurance plan? These doctors are not selling you a panacea; they are selling you a song and a dance. My mom was a victim of a similar scam perpetrated for years by a prominent New York dermatologist.

I know of a prominent surgeon on Long Island who is selling vitamins to women with breast cancer. I know this because a close friend, on whom he operated for breast cancer, was talked into purchasing these vitamins by the doctor himself. She felt pressured to purchase them after what she claimed was a very strong sell. "The vitamins were more potent and digestible than the ones you could buy in the store," he told her. So she purchased these vitamins for about $40 a bottle.

The night my friend called to tell me what happened, I asked her to read off the ingredients of the vitamins, and I was startled when she came across phytoestrogens. These are plant- (phyto-) derived estrogenlike hormones. There is no evidence that phytoestrogen supplementation in tablet form protects against breast cancer or is even safe. Furthermore (as explained in an article by Dr. J. Schwartz), concurrent use of high-dosage phytoestrogen supplements and tamoxifen in women with breast cancer should also be discouraged until further information is available, because of the potential for phytoestrogens to antagonize the desired antiestrogenic effects of tamoxifen.[10] And my friend was prescribed tamoxifen by the same team of doctors who sold her these vitamins. Fearful of saying anything to the surgeon (she depended on him for her postoperative care), she just threw the $40 bottle into the trash.

According to the California Medical Association legal department (taken from the *American Medical Association News*, June 7, 1999), physicians can be held liable for recommending products as remedies for conditions they are not trained to treat.[11] They can be found guilty of malpractice and possibly lose their licenses.

Because this thoroughly unprofessional practice has become endemic, the AMA ethics council issued a report in 1998 that strongly discouraged doctors from selling vitamins and other health-related, nonprescription products from their offices. But according the *AMA News,* the House of Delegates refused to approve it.[12]

Finally, in 1998, the ethics council of the AMA made the following statement. If you do sell such products, you must:

1. Make sure that any claims you make about the product are scientifically valid and are backed up by peer-reviewed literature and other unbiased scientific sources.
2. Disclose your financial interest in any product you sell.
3. Avoid monopolistic arrangements that hold patients captive. Encourage manufacturers to make products available through other channels, such as pharmacies, so that patients have a choice.

Should I Buy Something Sold on the Radio or TV?

I am sure people are still spending billions of dollars on potions and elixirs sold on radio and TV. Products promising weight loss and hair growth seem to be hotter than ever. Hollywood stars, or more likely has-beens, are out there promoting products that in most cases are never going to do what they tell you they will. So, I strongly recommend that if you see any medical product on an infomercial or advertised on your favorite radio talk show, don't waste your time or hard-earned money. Instead, turn to another station.

You have seen how a physician can change a simple $50 to $150 visit into one that costs well over $1,000. Rather than help you, however, such an expensive and frequently time-consuming visit may put you at greater risk. There are superbly talented, ethical, and kind physicians available to you in every area of expertise. I hope that what I have written will help you develop a knack for avoiding unscrupulous doctors and inappropriate care. I also hope that if you *have* been victimized by an unethical practitioner you will be motivated, after reading this chapter, to find a new one.

How can you avoid being taken in by one of the tricks of the trade?

1. Find a good doctor (see Chapter 1).
2. When you're in the hospital, ask the specialist why and how often he or she needs to see you.
3. If your aged or incapacitated relative is in the hospital, do not allow the doctor to call consultations without your approval.
4. Don't allow physicians to perform tests on you unless they are qualified. If you see they are cheating the system, leave the practice and report them to the state Office of Professional Misconduct (OPMC).
5. Never purchase vitamins or any other products at a doctor's office. I would suggest you leave that type of practice.
6. Read your insurance bills carefully and call the physician's office if you feel you have been overcharged. If you are dissatisfied with the response, report him to your insurance carrier—they might investigate.
7. Before any surgery or before any chemotherapy, get a second opinion.

8. If you need to get a drug at your doctor's office, ask for a unit dose, usually in a single-use prefilled syringe. Make sure you are shown the unopened syringe.

9. Get all your blood tests at an outside lab. Rare exceptions include an urgent INR (for patients who take warfarin) and a finger stick sugar.

10. Don't go to physicians who don't accept your insurance.

11. Even if your insurance carrier paid in full for a test or a consult or the ten unnecessary hospital visits, you still ought to report the doctors to the insurance company. Patients are sometimes just as guilty as the unscrupulous doctors in causing the health-insurance rates in this country to keep rising ever higher.

CHAPTER 4

Should I Get
a Second Opinion?

My question for you is a simple one: Why *not* get a second opinion? In most cases, it doesn't cost you anything. Your insurance company will usually pay for it. I'm not necessarily talking about basic care here. You should be able to trust your doctor with all that. (If you ever have reason to doubt his or her judgment about something simple and straightforward, however, get another doctor pronto.) But if you are going for a special procedure or for surgery, then why not ask for a second opinion? The stakes are just too high. And the old adage "two heads are better than one" is a good one. Of course, a differing second opinion can create a predicament. Who, after all, is right? In that circumstance, I suggest that the patient ask the two physicians with differing views to confer and perhaps arrive at a mutual opinion. If this is not possible, you might have to make that decision (albeit at this point an educated one) yourself, or you can go on and request a third opinion.

In my practice I have never been upset when a patient has requested a second opinion. Actually, in complicated cases, I have often asked for a second opinion myself. If your physician is offended by your request, then perhaps you should choose another doctor. You never want to suffer as a result of any one physician's bias or, worse, as a result of his or her arrogance or presumed infallibility. This sort of hubris, which is admittedly such a common human failing in people from all different walks of life, can be downright dangerous when it comes to physicians.

The best way to make my point is to recount a handful of cases either known to me or in which I had some direct involvement. As you will see, there are patients who refused either to get a second opinion or to believe what they were told when they did, and who suffered untoward consequences because of it. Other times, patients who had reason to question the first diagnosis they received benefited greatly by seeking out a second opinion that turned out to be the right one.

When I was training to become a cardiologist, I was called to see a young man who appeared to have had a large heart attack several days before. He was in the ICU of a city hospital and clearly very sick, but because he had not come to the hospital immediately—not for several days, actually—we were unable to determine if he indeed had had a heart attack.

Two of the brightest attending physicians at the hospital were in charge of the case, though neither was a cardiologist. After due deliberation, these brilliant but also arrogant men declared that the patient had an unusual viral infection of the heart called myocarditis, but that he did not have coronary artery disease. I suggested to both doctors that they might indeed be right about the myocarditis, but that this young man also had coronary artery disease and that if we didn't act on it the results would be catastrophic. I brought my attending in to speak to them, and even though he agreed with my diagnosis and suppositions, he seemed indifferent or too timid to persuade the men to reconsider their strongly held opinion.

When you are in a city-run hospital, you don't get second opinions. You get the doctor who is assigned to you. Period. Well, after I made it clear to all of them that I thought it was a potentially grave error not to send this patient for an angiogram to make certain he didn't have coronary disease, I was told by both the senior attendings that I was no longer part of the case. Remember what I said about hubris. They had convinced not only themselves but also the resident doctors in training that this patient had an unusual infection and not a heart attack.

As it turns out, the patient did indeed have coronary disease. He had a second heart attack shortly thereafter and died. I remember the resident doctors paging me urgently and asking me to run over to see the patient whom they had diagnosed incorrectly, but at that point there was nothing we could do. The autopsy confirmed severe coronary disease. The two senior attendings circulated articles to the staff about rare viruses and how they can sometimes cause coronary disease, but they never apologized to me or, more important, to the patient's wife and family.

Nothing ever came of this episode. No legal action was taken. But it taught me a profound lesson that I have kept with me to this day. A physician must treat his or her patients without arrogance and without preconceived notions or bias when considering all possible diagnoses. I have not spoken to either physician since.

In municipal hospitals and in most veterans' hospitals, too, there usually isn't a procedure that allows a patient to obtain a second opinion. However, in most other hospital settings, getting a second opinion is quite easy. I would suggest that you not ask your physician about who might be best for a second opinion, but instead ask the residents in training or nurses who they would recommend. Remember, if you are already in the hospital, your choices are somewhat limited. It might also be politically difficult for a physician to disagree openly with his colleague. Thus, if you are having any elective surgery, I urge you to get your second opinion before you enter the hospital and from a physician not affiliated with the same hospital.

For the past ten years I've offered to provide a free second opinion for all my friends and family, and at times, for friends of my family. So I've given quite a few second opinions.

About eight years ago, my grandfather, then well into his eighties, told his doctor he frequently experienced pressure in his stomach and chest after he ate and often belched while walking on the golf course. When his physician told him not to worry, that it was just gas or a minor stomach problem, and prescribed over-the-counter Maalox for his condition, he knew enough to call me. After listening to him for several minutes, I came to the conclusion that Gramps probably had severe coronary disease. Even though his symptoms were an unusual manifestation of this condition, I felt he needed attention right away. Shortly thereafter he underwent an angiogram. To this day, it remains the most abnormal study I've ever seen. The main artery was about 90 percent blocked, and the right artery was completely occluded. It's a miracle he didn't die out there on the golf course.

Gramps survived his angiogram and his bypass surgery and returned to his normal life.

Seven years later, on what was his ninetieth birthday, in front of all his family and friends, he thanked me for saving his life. I have rarely felt so honored or felt such a sense of purpose in my life.

More recently, a friend of my father's had an unnecessary stress test prior to a very minor surgical procedure. Although the doctor interpreted the stress test as showing no evidence for coronary disease, he did note that the patient had three extra beats in a row as he finished his exercise. I'm not sure why, since this is truly not a meaningful or disturbing symptom, but he sent him to a very busy heart center to see an arrhythmia expert. This expert should have told him not to worry, but instead scheduled him for a very invasive and complex study to determine if he needed a pacemaker or defibrillator.

Now, my father's friend is a smart man, and as this situation began to balloon out of control, he had the sense to get a second opinion. With his records in hand, he and I carefully reviewed his stress test. Everything looked normal to me. Then I called the heart doctor who had performed the stress test. I asked a few questions, and after listening to his answers I realized that his opinion was incorrect. We then called the heart-center doctor, who sent us his evaluation. In this doctor's evaluation he erroneously noted that the patient had a history of a heart attack and that the patient complained of palpitations. (According to the patient, he had no symptoms.)

I think the first physician was just not a very well informed and had mistakenly sent my father's friend for a consultation that he did not require. I doubt this physician was part of a large scheme to fleece him, but the arrhythmia "expert" at the famous heart hospital, well, in my view, his actions were inappropriate. Thankfully, in this case, a second opinion prevented this mess from going any further, but I'm sure that there are many others who get caught up in this doctor's dangerous game.

I have a friend and medical colleague who sometimes sends us patients to evaluate. One night about twelve years ago he called me in distress to say that his mom had been admitted to a small local hospital with early gangrene of her toes. An angiogram had been done, and the doctors there told the woman and her two sons that both of her legs would probably need to be amputated. Needless to say, the entire family was in a state of near shock.

Even in those early days of my practice I followed a simple rule: Get a second opinion and get it at a center of excellence. Although I didn't have all the information, I did know I had to act fast for the sake of my friend and colleague's mother. So I immediately called the vascular specialists at Montefiore Medical Center and had her transferred there that night.

Upon examination, her legs unquestionably showed severe hematomas and very cool, ulcerated toes. But amputation was out of the question. In an operation I was to learn is fairly routine, the Montefiore surgeons were able to open both arteries and increase the flow of blood in both of her legs and feet. I am happy to report that she remains on both of her feet to this day. But if her sons had not called me and I had not called a real specialist, the consequences would have been devastating. She might have had to endure a double amputation, been wheelchair-bound for life, and probably would have suffered an early death.

The only time I have actually agreed that a patient should file a malpractice suit against his doctor occurred after I was called upon for a second opinion regarding his need for a pacemaker. Actually he had already received a second opinion from another cardiologist, but since that doctor just reviewed his records, never examined the gentleman, and also came to the same conclusion—that he get a pacemaker—the patient decided to come see me.

The patient did not need a pacemaker, but as part of my exam I noticed that this gentleman had a mass adjacent to an inverted nipple on his right breast. His original cardiologist, who had been treating him for two years, apparently had never examined his right breast, my guess being because the heart is on the *left* side. Anyway, the patient turned out to have breast cancer (which, by the way, had nothing to do with his slow heart rate) and required a mastectomy and extensive chemotherapy. More than six years later, he is still without that pacemaker.

Sometimes even doctors need to consider a second opinion about matters concerning their own health. In February 2003, a seasoned physician whom I've known for many years went to a local emergency room with a tearing and annoying chest pain after lifting a heavy trunk. The emergency-room doctor told him that his EKG was fine and that he could go home, that he had probably just pulled a muscle. It might please you to learn that this patient refused to go home. Convinced that the ER doctor was missing something, and deeply suspicious that something was very wrong inside his chest, he demanded that he be seen by a cardiologist and that he be admitted at least until the appropriate tests were completed and showed him to be in good health. In spite of the ER doctor's skepticism and vocal reluctance to grant his wishes, the doctor/patient was eventually admitted.

The next morning a cardiology resident examined the doctor and told him he was fine. Not until 3:00 P.M., and only after both he and his wife complained bitterly, did the resident return with the attending cardiologist. Neither doctor could explain this tearing pain, but both told him it was not his heart. A chest X ray, bloods, and an echo were done, and he was told that they were normal. The cardiologist thought perhaps it was his gallbladder and called a general surgeon to see him. He too remarked that it was nothing. With four doctors' unanimous opinions that he was fine, he was discharged and sent home.

At work the next day he and a few of his fellow MDs got together for their usual coffee in the solarium at the local hospital. And as he told his story about this tearing chest pain, which in fact was still annoying him, one of his old friends remarked that it sounded like an aortic dissection. That's a life-threatening tear in the aorta. So four seasoned doctors halted their coffee klatch and headed downstairs to the radiologist to get a CAT scan. The scan revealed what could have been deadly: a tear along the entire three-foot length of the aorta. He might well have died the previous night in his bed at home or the night before that in the hospital. He was immediately transferred to a medical center in New York City and emergency surgery was performed at once.

The doctor recovered and is doing well now, but he asked me recently how not one but four physicians could have missed the correct diagnosis. His symptoms were classic, but not one of the doctors had taken a careful history. The ER doctor, you will re-call, had wanted to send him home right away. No one examined all his pulses, a thirty-second exam that probably would have alerted any one of them to this serious and life-threatening problem. In the end, it was his coffee buddies, who had the pa-tience to listen to his story in a careful and unbiased fashion, who made the right diagnosis.

If you are a patient with a serious health issue and your sur-geon begins telling you about the newest, latest, and greatest surgical technique, the alarm bells should go off right away about the absolute necessity of getting a second opinion. *Newest, latest, and greatest* might mean the procedure is so new that the surgeon hasn't done many of them, and we all know that prac-tice makes perfect. No need to be a guinea pig, right? Here's a real-life example.

Mr. M is a powerful and fit seventy-five-year-old man. He was admitted to a hospital in Florida with severe coronary disease and a leak in his aortic valve. The cardiac surgeon there extolled the virtues of the newest type of surgery in his field, known these days as minimally invasive bypass or beating-heart sur-gery. The potential advantages were thought to be a reduction in what doctors call neurocognitive impairment, i.e., a potential re-duction in the risk of stroke, and in a post-op complication that results in patients being less smart or quick-witted than they were before they went on the heart-lung machine. Also, in the-ory, a decreased hospital stay, because the patient is never placed on a heart-lung machine. The disadvantage is that the heart is beating—not still—and the field of view is drastically reduced for the surgeon. In addition, you cannot operate on the aortic valve in a beating heart. Needless to say, Mr. M did not get a second opinion.

During surgery, the doctor bypassed three arteries and "decided" that the leak in the aortic valve was not severe enough to fix, though we already know that he could not have attempted to repair it while doing the surgery the "latest and greatest" way.

Shortly after recovering from the operation, the patient returned with chest pain and severe heart failure. Two of the bypasses were closed (most likely the result of technical problems), and the valve leak, only a few months later (when I reviewed it anyway), was quite severe. These complications might have been prevented if Mr. M had had the surgery the old-fashioned way on the heart-lung machine.

About two years after his first surgery, Mr. M underwent a second procedure, this time electing for old-fashioned bypass surgery (by another surgeon). He had his aortic valve replaced and two of the grafts redone. The risk of death from the second surgery was perhaps three times the risk of the first, but lucky for him, he pulled through it.

Sometimes, thanks to coincidence or luck, a patient gets a second opinion without actually having sought one. Since I trained in mostly large university hospitals, it was not until my first year of practice that I came to realize what small community hospitals were all about. What I found there would taint my opinion of these wannabe institutions for the rest of my life. In exchange for the privilege of admitting our patients to a local community hospital, my partner and I were asked to teach the students and interns there. Although many of the patients had run-of-the-mill medical problems, we did see some unusual cardiac patients there.

One was Mr. Mulligan, a proud, funny Irishman with a great laugh and sweet smile. He worked as the doorman for a well-known multimillionaire in the early 1990s, and from the moment I met him I liked the man. He had come to the hospital complaining of chest pains. When these pains occurred in the hospital ICU, however, he developed ventricular tachycardia and only survived after he was shocked back to life. He did not have a heart attack but something called unstable angina (periods of lack of oxygen to the heart not severe enough to cause immediate heart damage) and what would have been death from the arrhythmia, caused by the lack of blood flow to the heart.

Common sense would tell you that this man needed to have an angiogram and have his artery opened before he "died" again. But the doctor he was assigned to decided to send him out of the ICU and then for a stress test. You probably think I am joking, but I am not. Every time he has chest pain, he "dies," and this doctor is sending him for a stress test.

When he left the ICU, he was put under my care. I was a new attending, green and still wet behind the ears. And I was being watched by many of the doctors who, frankly, did not want a sharp, young heart doctor in their institution. But I also had to do the best I could for the patient. So without obtaining the senior cardiologist's permission, I canceled the patient's transfer from the ICU, canceled the stress test, put him on potent blood thinners, and transferred him right away to another hospital for an urgent cardiac catheterization.

His badly clogged artery was opened up that day with a balloon catheter. Shortly thereafter, the senior doctors decided that I would not be allowed to see the cardiology service patients (I guess they were offended when I changed their orders) who had already been seen by the ICU cardiologist. I had hoped to continue my voluntary care and teaching of medicine, but after I was told I could only see certain patients, I withdrew my offer.

A small price to pay, right? For twelve years, Mr. Mulligan and I have joked about his good fortune and how he might not have ever seen or known seen his grandchildren had he not gotten a chance second opinion from a fledgling physician.

Here's another example of what I mean. About five years ago, a middle-aged woman was given a diagnosis of uterine cancer by a local surgeon and scheduled for a hysterectomy. Since she had lost over thirty pounds in the preceding two months, she was told that the tumor had most likely spread and that at the very least she would need chemotherapy to prolong her life. Lucky for her the patient's preoperative cardiogram noted an irregular rhythm, and the surgery was delayed, at least until she could see a cardiologist. She happened to pick me.

When she came to my office I saw a very anxious woman who was suffering from pronounced weight loss and an irregular, fast heartbeat. Even her eyes were bulging. Do you remember the comedian Marty Feldman? What I saw before me was a textbook case of hyperthyroidism (an overactive thyroid). So before examining her I asked her to put out her hands, watched the fine tremor (which she told me had started just a few months ago), and told her I might have good news.

With her family now seated beside her I told her that all of her symptoms were probably just from hyperthyroidism and that the mass in her uterus, whether cancer or just a fibroid tumor, was not causing her symptoms. We canceled her scheduled hysterectomy. Two days later the lab confirmed the diagnosis of hyperthyroidism. After treatment her heart rate returned to normal, her tremor subsided, and she regained her strength and weight. The tumor ended up just being a fibroid, a noncancerous growth. Had she gone in for the operation with undiagnosed hyperthyroidism, she might have developed a devastating type of illness, known as thyroid storm, and died. Fate works in strange ways, doesn't it?

Always remember the following when you consider a second opinion:

1. I wholeheartedly recommend a second opinion when any dangerous operation or procedure is contemplated.
2. I would suggest you tell your physician before he or she renders a decision that you plan on obtaining two opinions regarding your care.
3. Get a new doctor if your physician seems upset about it.
4. Try to get the second opinion before you enter the hospital and get it from a physician not affiliated with that same hospital.
5. If the physicians should disagree in their diagnosis, ask them to provide literature to support their decision. Then ask your regular medical doctor to help you make the final decision.

CHAPTER 5

Should I Take Part in a Scientific Study?

In my opinion there are many more risks than benefits for anyone considering enrolling in a clinical study. If there are reasonable medications or procedures of proven efficacy available to
you, then why should you or a member of your family serve as a
guinea pig in a clinical investigation of a new drug or therapy?
Unless you truly have a terminal illness and all other options have
been tried and proven useless, I would never advise you to join a
study. In this chapter I will review the numerous risks inherent in
these trials and give examples of some studies gone wrong.

The first fundamental fact that you many not be aware of is
that most physicians who are engaged in these studies are paid
thousands of dollars for each new patient they manage to enroll.
As has been noted in a recent article from the prestigious *Journal of the American Medical Association:*

> The stakes in clinical testing of new drugs and devices are
> high because for-profit corporations stand to gain large

revenues from marketing new products before their competitors. Therefore, the rapid recruitment of sufficient numbers of patients has become paramount and may explain why manufacturers are willing to offer investigators $2000 to $5000 per patient in certain cases, in contrast to $1000 per subject enrolled in NIH-sponsored studies. Regardless of whether these payments, in fact, represent usual and customary or ordinary payments, they do represent reimbursements several-fold greater than those of Medicare or third-party carriers and explain why they are sought by both academic investigators and community-based practitioners. There are other informative articles on this subject as well.[2, 3]

(A detailed review of the pharmaceutical industry and its practices is outlined in Chapter 6.)

As you can no doubt imagine, some physicians employed by a hospital depend on this revenue to keep their job, much as academics must bring in grant money in order to keep theirs. Many are offered paid speaking engagements by the pharmaceutical companies to lecture or "brainwash" other physicians into participating in a study. Of course the lecture might be in a place like Aspen, an hour or so before a great afternoon of skiing, with all expenses paid for everyone.

For example, I recently spoke to a heart-failure expert employed by a major university who told me with not a little pride that he almost doubled his income by giving lectures to physicians at restaurants and resorts sponsored by rival pharmaceutical companies. So you must consider the obvious bias that the doctor/investigator brings to his attempts to get you to enroll in his study.

Finally, and perhaps unbelievably, our own FDA often hires the same physicians who are being paid to conduct trials for a pharmaceutical company to decide whether that same drug should be approved for release to the general public. In fact, a study by *USA Today* found that 54 percent of the experts (usually physicians) hired to advise the government on the safety and effectiveness of medicine have financial relationships with the pharmaceutical companies that will be helped or hurt by their decisions.[4] The physician's bias, therefore, may be so deeply ingrained that without even realizing it, the investigator may be violating his oath of a doctor: Do no harm.

The first thing you should ask yourself before entering any study is *Why should I?* For example, why enroll yourself in a double-blind study (a study where neither you nor your physician knows what medication you are getting) for an illness (like hypertension, diabetes, angina, or especially a heart attack) when there are already very good medications to treat you? Why knowingly take that sort of risk with your very life? There were patients, for example, perhaps some who are reading these pages for the first time, who participated in clinical trials for Posicor, which made it to market for a short while but which interacted with other drugs and may have killed several patients from arrhythmias, or for Rezulin, which also made it briefly to market but which killed several patients and made others very ill from associated liver toxicity. I can assure you that none of them would do it again.

In a Pulitzer Prize–winning article published in *The Los Angeles Times*, the author, David Willman, reviews the horrible process in which Posicor was approved by the FDA—in spite of 143 sudden deaths![5] The interesting part of this article describes how the FDA advisory committee chairman—Dr. Barry Massie—was also a coinvestigator of a Posicor drug trial (sponsored by the pharmaceutical company Roche). And although he recused himself in the final vote to recommend approval of the drug (the drug won approval by a vote of five to three), there remained an obvious conflict of interest. To make the situation perhaps even more troubling is the fact that Roche hired him as a speaker for the drug and even released information that "quoted Massie to buttress the company's claim that 'the incidence of side effects was low' during clinical studies of Posicor." When confronted with these ties, Massie told the reporter, "'You do wonder how the world would perceive it. I'm glad I didn't vote, let's put it that way.'"

During my fellowship in cardiology (a training program after my residency in medicine), there were many successful trials for the clot-busting drugs, called thrombolytics, used for the treatment of acute myocardial infarction (heart attack). Yet there was one study of patients with unstable angina (patients with resting chest pain but without evidence of a heart attack) in which I and many of my fellow colleagues refused to enroll our patients. Why? Quite simple. Only a few years before, a study using a simple blood thinner called heparin was shown to be very effective in preventing heart attack and death in patients with unstable angina and did not possess the most dangerous risk of thrombolytics, which is intracranial bleeding (sudden uncontrollable bleeding in your brain). Because the pharmaceutical companies and the lead investigators had trouble enrolling patients in the study, they went as far as sending letters to these doctors in training stating that they would pay $100 for every patient the doctors enrolled. When the study was eventually completed and the data presented in *The Journal of the American Heart Association* (*Circulation*) in 1994, it was shown that intracranial hemorrhage occurred in 0.55 percent of the thrombolysis patients and in not one from the heparin group. In the end the authors of the study concluded that the drug was "not beneficial and may even be harmful."[6] I am proud to say we made the right decision.

I should also point out here that most cardiologists would almost certainly agree that if someone is having a large heart attack (called an ST-elevation heart attack, since that is the way it looks on the cardiogram), the best way to treat it is not with drugs but with a surgical procedure that opens up the closed vessel with a catheter and an angioplasty balloon or a coronary stent. In fact, in a clinician update article in *Circulation*, the authors state that emergency percutaneous coronary intervention (PCI) without thrombolytics therapy has been shown to offer a substantial benefit over thrombolytic therapy. The authors note that these benefits include a significant reduction in mortality even in spite of the potential delay that patients have when they go to the catheterization lab (for PCI) to get their artery opened.[7, 8] Yet, even so, newer types of thrombolytics are still being studied to determine if they can be as effective as the catheter method or used in situations where the catheter method (PCI) is not available.

The investigators carrying out these trials will seek to prove that these newer drugs do not have a risk of life-threatening bleeding (even these same investigators note a 0.9 percent risk of intracranial hemorrhage—a bleed into your brain—associated with fibrinolytic therapy) as high as that of the old ones.[9] They also argue, in defense of the experimental drugs, that not all heart-attack victims are situated close enough to hospitals that perform PCIs. I dispute this last assertion vigorously, since studies have shown that you are better off taking a half-hour ambulance ride for a PCI than taking a thrombolytic.[10–13]

And what really bothers me is that most of these studies are being done in hospitals that perform PCIs. In a study called TIMI 31 (Thrombolysis in Myocardial Infarction), which is being funded by the manufacturer British Biotech, researchers are treating heart-attack patients with one of four different-sized doses of a thrombolytic, the largest being five times greater than the smallest. Sixty minutes after administration of the drug, you are sent for an angiogram to determine what the given dose has achieved.[14] In other words, you *will* be getting the preferred treatment. Not because it might save your life, mind you, but because it will enable the researchers to measure the efficacy of the different dosages of the drug and open up the artery with a catheter just in case the drug doesn't work. But common sense as well as clinical data (70 percent of all bleeds occur at the site of vascular punctures) says that placing a catheter in your artery after any thrombolytic increases your risk of bleeding complications at that site.[15]

In fact, the investigator's description of this trial states that "the TIMI 31 is a phase II, open-label, multi-center, dose escalation study to determine the efficacy, safety, tolerability, pharmacokinetics, and pharmacodynamics of BB-10153 in ST Segment Elevation myocardial infarction."[16] In other words, the main object of the study is not only to see if the drug works, but to see if it is safe (i.e., that it does not cause deadly bleeds in your brain) and if it is well tolerated.

So here you are, having a heart attack, when a nurse and doctor come down to the emergency room and ask you to enroll in their new thrombolytic study. Your investigating physicians would in effect be experimenting on you to see if too large a dose causes you to bleed to death or too small a dose has no impact whatsoever, when they're aware that the best treatment is an elevator ride away.

In the university hospital where I work I asked ten cardiologists if they would participate as patients in a study that would give them a clot-opening drug instead of going immediately for a PCI. All ten of them told me they would unquestionably opt for the PCI technique.

In defense of the study, a safer and more potent drug is needed, particularly in areas where there isn't a cath lab ready and willing to open up the artery that's causing a heart attack. But the excuse given to me by two prominent investigators— that patients enrolled in the study get VIP treatment and go to the lab much faster than the average patient having an MI— bothers me. It suggests that most patients having life-threatening heart attacks do not get the fastest and best care.

In the 1980s, powerful drugs called antiarrhythmics were being developed in an effort to prevent dangerous arrhythmias in patients with heart disease. A notorious trial called the Cardiac Arrhythmia Suppression Trial (CAST) was begun with patients who had some isolated extra beats after their heart attack to see what the effect of these drugs would be.[17] Meanwhile, the

FDA approved one of the drugs (Encainide) before this trial was over, and the data was thoroughly investigated. The heart experts in the hospital I trained in refused to be part of the study (citing stories from their colleagues who had used the drugs), since they felt they were dangerous. Sure enough, instead of stopping the arrhythmias, there were many case reports that showed that these drugs often started dangerous arrhythmias, even killed people. Even as the study continued, my colleagues and I saw patients admitted to our hospital with strange and life-threatening incessant arrhythmias that seemed to be caused by these drugs and by encainide in particular, since thanks to the FDA it had already been approved for sale. I remember the salespeople for the company that manufactured encainide taking us to lunch and pleading with us to use this product. Finally, in 1989, the results of the CAST trial were released. They showed that patients who took encainide were 1.5 times more likely to die than those who took nothing.[18] Days later the drug was withdrawn from the market. No one knows how many people were needlessly killed during this time period by encainide.

You would think that after that trial no reasonable person would enroll as a patient in a trial of an antiarrhythmic agent after a heart attack. That wasn't the case when the Survival with Oral D-Sotalol (SWORD) study began.[19] This time, however, my hospital was involved with the trial. In general, doctors involved in these big trials have special nurses go through charts to see if any of their patients are eligible candidates. (Most patients do not realize that they sign a piece of paper when they are admitted to the hospital that permits the hospital to make these evaluations.) Two of my patients fit the admission criteria, and the nurse called me and asked if they could be enrolled. I said no. Soon I was being harassed by some of the physicians involved in the trial and deemed uncooperative. Research is important to maintain our hospital's esteem in the community, I was told. However, the SWORD study was terminated prematurely because the patients who received the drug were almost twice as likely to die as those who did not.[20]

I am not saying absolutely that you should never, ever take part in a study, however. For example, clinical studies on heart failure have often produced great results, in particular studies on beta-blockers and angiotensin-converting enzyme inhibitors (ACEIs).

But there is a caveat here as well. In the United States there are now eight ACE inhibitors that have been approved for the treatment of heart failure and high blood pressure. The most important study that showed their benefit in treating and preventing heart failure is called the CONSENSUS study (Cooperative Northern Scandinavian Enalapril Survival Study). Published in 1987, this study demonstrated a 40 percent reduction in mortality at six months in patients with severe heart failure who were already on standard therapy. In studies like this, one patient gets the drug (in this case enalapril); the other gets a placebo (sugar pill). Neither the patient nor the physician knows which patient is getting the actual medication (called a double-blind study). This study was very important, since it showed that medications like enalapril save lives.[21]

In the years that followed, other pharmaceutical companies conducted numerous other studies to make their case that their particular ACEI drug (called a copycat drug) also saved lives. In general, they all came to the same conclusion: ACEI drugs save lives in patients with congestive heart failure. Great, right? Well, how about those patients who participated in these studies who were given the sugar pill? They didn't do too well, did they? In general, when compared to the patients who refused enrollment in the study and who then took another ACEI drug, those who participated in the study and received placebo were much more likely to die or to become sicker. Consequently, I would never enroll in a study that is conducted to prove that a copycat drug is as effective as the drug that is already available!

Always ask the researcher who wishes to enroll you in a study if there are any similar medications available, and if there are, tell him or her to go away. Other examples of copycat drug studies (and thus similar trials) are those that were conducted for the stomach drugs similar to Prilosec (the original drug in that field), which include AcipHex and Prevacid. In these cases, patient's ulcers may not have healed as well as they would have if they had been given the drug already available, Prilosec.

These double-blind trials of new drugs that have the same effect as other drugs of proven efficacy are thoroughly immoral in my view. A recent trial by Merck (the RENAAL trial) found that a drug named Cozaar (losartan), an angiotensin receptor blocker (ARB) that acts in a manner similar to that of the ACEIs, protected kidney function as well as the ACEI drugs did.[22] It did not, however, reduce cardiovascular death as significantly as an ACEI called ramipril did (HOPE Study).[23] In addition, those patients who received placebos were not offered an ACEI and thus received substandard care.

At the time of this study, the American Diabetes Association strongly recommended the use of an ACEI in all diabetics with hypertension. And while the results of this study were indeed very important since they do strongly show that drugs like losartan can be an important (though more expensive than the generic ACEI) agent in the prevention of kidney failure in diabetics (in fact, this was the first major trial in what we call type 2 diabetics), I remain concerned for those study patients who received a placebo. None of the patients enrolled in the placebo group received an ACEI, even though a very well-known study published back in 1993 showed ACEIs to be of such significant benefit (again in type 1 diabetic patients) that these authors proposed "that this therapy be used in normotensive and hypertensive patients with diabetes [note that the authors did not distinguish between what type of diabetes in their conclusion] and clinically evident nephropathy."[24] In fact, the RENAAL study was discontinued early, not because of the obvious benefit of losartan but because the doctors in charge of the study made the conclusions that "based on new evidence that ACEIs, which were excluded by design from the study, may be effective in reducing the incidence of cardiovascular events in patients with renal impairment."[25]

My guess is that the authors were talking about the HOPE trial, submitted for publication in that month, which showed the significant benefit of ACEI.[26] Essentially, patients who got the placebo received substandard care (based on the data I have shown you as well as the American Diabetes Association recommendations). Perhaps they did so for the future benefit of other patients, but I have to wonder about the possible incentive some of the physicians had, since the study was paid for by Merck.

It is a sad fact of life that physicians and pharmaceutical companies are more than willing to withhold life-saving treatment from half of their study participants, sometimes making millions and possibly billions of dollars at the expense of these human beings who got nothing except increases in morbidity and mortality. Therefore, the first question a patient should ask before considering any enrollment in a study is whether there are medications available to the patient that are similar to the one in the study, and if so, what are the known benefits of that drug? Frankly, I wonder how any physician could play a game of Russian roulette with his patient, but this is exactly what some physicians are doing.

As an example I would like to use a type of drug that was given to patients with heart failure during the 1980s and well into the 1990s. Milrinone, amrinone, enoximone, vesnarinone, and pimobendan are all drugs that increase the beating of the heart by inhibiting a special enzyme known as phosphodiesterase III. These drugs also have something else in common: tragic consequences resulting from their use. In large clinical trials on patients with heart failure that were conducted over the course of more than ten years, each of these drugs resulted in an increase in deaths for those unfortunate patients who were enrolled in the studies and received the studies' drugs instead of the harmless placebo. Some of the death rates were so significant that the trial was stopped well before the desired number of patients had even been enrolled.[27]

As described above, there are types of drugs that are repeatedly studied (in real patients versus a placebo) in spite of their lack of benefit or in spite of the fact that they can cause harm and even death. In this case, despite overwhelming evidence that drugs that make weak hearts beat stronger increased mortality, for year after year patients were enrolled in study after study of new drugs that increased the heart's strength. To date, there is not a single drug that increases the heart's strength (contractility) that does not also increase mortality. (Perhaps the only exception would be foxglove, known as digoxin, which was described by William Withering in 1785. Data from large randomized trials do show that digoxin often makes patients with heart failure feel better and probably does not increase their mortality.)

A blood thinner known as warfarin (or Coumadin) was shown to prevent stroke in patients with an irregular heart rhythm known as atrial fibrillation. In spite of the obvious results, several other huge trials of the drug, each of which enrolled thousands of patients, were either repeated by different institutions or not stopped prematurely (to their credit, Canadian investigators did stop their trial prematurely when they saw overwhelming evidence that warfarin did prevent stroke in patients with atrial fibrillation). Consequently, one could argue that many patients who received a placebo or even aspirin were ill served, and some of those patients who did suffer a stroke might not have if they had received warfarin.[28-33]

Randomized trials remain the standard by which promising medical therapies are evaluated. Not too long ago medications were used on the assumption that they were beneficial. Today these studies provide absolute evidence of the efficacy of drugs and devices for the treatment of often life-threatening illnesses.

So there is no question that these studies need to continue and have been responsible for the prolongation of millions of lives.

It is my belief, however, that patient consent is often not truly informed ("read this, sign here") and that many patients are persuaded by hospital staff who have financial incentives (through grants and payments from pharmaceutical companies) to enroll patients. Studies are often duplicated (at the expense of the patient) to see if a similar drug works as well as one available or to determine if it has other serious side effects. After years of developing a drug only to see similar drugs cause harm, pharmaceutical companies seem to continue trials in the hope that their drug might be different. You have just read about an example of this. Of course the written consent does not say anything about the fact that drugs similar to the one you may be given have increased deaths by 100 percent or that if you enroll in this study you may not receive a medication that is already considered a standard of care or, finally, that your physician will be receiving $5,000 if you enroll in this trial.

With the above in mind, these are my suggestions.

1. If there are other effective medications available, never enroll in a study.
2. Especially avoid studies that are in a phase I or phase II stage. These types of trials are more interested in finding out if the drug is safe and at what dose it might work or result in a dangerous outcome.
3. Find out if there have been similar studies in the past and what the results of these studies have been.

4. Office-based drug studies are usually an ingenious method for the pharmaceutical company to give money to your doctor. In fact, sometimes the drugs used are old drugs that were studied years ago. Don't enroll in them.

5. Ask your physician what he or she is paid to enroll you in the study and why he or she is involved.

6. Read the consent form very carefully. (It is required that you be told the potential risks and benefits.)

7. Ask an impartial physician his or her opinion.

8. Never enroll in any study when you are not given at least a few days to think about it.

9. Do not respond to any radio or television ads, even if you'll be paid to enroll in the study.

CHAPTER 6

The Pharmaceutical Industry

In a perfect world, the ideal pharmaceutical company—a Merck, a Pfizer, a Bristol-Myers Squibb—would create nothing but useful, affordable, sometimes life-saving products that satisfy the customer's every medical need, whether it be to reduce blood pressure or the level of cholesterol or even to heighten the sexual endurance of those who have found their performance somehow lacking. Indeed, over the past twenty years, there has been a bounty of wonder drugs and surgical devices that have improved and prolonged the lives of many. But as we know all too well, the real goal of any pharmaceutical company that survives in this day and age is to invent, develop, gain approval for, and market on a worldwide basis new drugs that generate maximum revenue and profits for the company and, in turn, for the company's shareholders. It is nothing more or less than the American way.

But as consumers of all the myriad products put before us by the makers of cereal or automobiles or household wares, we know that we do not always buy the most nutritious box of oatmeal or the safest car or the most powerful vacuum cleaner on the market. More often than not, and for better or worse, we buy the one that has been most cleverly and repeatedly advertised and marketed.

It should come as no surprise, then, that the rules of the capitalist workplace apply equally well to the pharmaceutical industry. A physician's choice may not necessarily be about which drug is best or cheapest, or which is just right for a particular patient's medical issue and metabolism. What it really comes down to, in the end, is often successful *marketing*. And that is also the problem: the way these companies market their products to patients and the physicians who prescribe them, and the mind-boggling costs that go along with these marketing efforts.

For example, in 2002 a report released by a nonprofit, nonpartisan consumer-health organization, Families USA, noted that on average the nine largest publicly traded U.S. pharmaceutical companies spent a total of $45.4 billion on marketing, advertising, and administration and only $19.1 billion on research and development for the year 2001. They found that "eight of the nine companies spent more than twice as much on marketing, advertising, and administration as they did on R&D."[1]

Figures published by IMS Health, Integrated Promotions Services, go even further in revealing just how much money is spent by these companies on promotion alone. In 2001 total promotional spending by all pharmaceutical companies was $19.059 billion. Of this, over $10 billion was spent on samples, $4.789 billion on office promotions (drug reps and their expenses), $702 million on hospital promotion (hospital reps and their expenses),

Company	Percent of Revenues Spent on Marketing/Advertising/Administration*
Merck	13
Pfizer	35
Bristol-Myers Squibb	27
Abbott Laboratories	23
Wyeth	37
Pharmacia	44
Eli Lilly	30
Schering-Plough	36
Allergan	42

www.familiesusa.org

$425 million on journal advertising, and $2.679 billion on direct marketing to the consumer (television, radio, newspapers, etc.).[2] Imagine if these companies spent only half as much money on these efforts. Imagine the reduction in cost that could be realized and the savings for consumers, not to mention the insurance industry.

The problematic relationship between the pharmaceutical industry and the health-care industry is so complex that I have broken this chapter into several parts. In the first part, I will discuss the marketing and/or the manipulation of the physician by the pharmaceutical representative. In the second part of the chapter, I will discuss how the different companies attempt to coerce the hospitals into using their medication over that of their competitors. I will then discuss the financial ties many physicians conducting clinical research have with the industry, and I will site specific examples of duplicitous behavior. Finally, I will defend the industry against the onslaught of gluttonous lawyers who have contributed to the high cost of medications to the consumer.

As I have already noted, the pharmaceutical industry spends billions of dollars per year marketing its products. Part of this effort is carried out by a national force of sales representatives. For the most part these reps are young men and women, college-educated, though often *without any background* in medicine, who are sent to doctors' offices all over the country to "educate" physicians about the company's offering of drugs and to provide samples of same for his or her patients.

In the Merck Annual Report for 2000, the company writes that the "company's professional representatives communicate the effectiveness, safety and value of our products to health care professionals in private practice, group practices, and managed care organizations."[3] In congressional hearings on the industry's practices, industry representatives reiterated that these reps do indeed play an important role in educating physicians and in providing samples to patients who may not be able to obtain the medication in a timely manner.

I would suggest that a more honest appraisal of the reps' role should be worded as follows: The company's professional representatives frequently communicate half-truths and exaggerate the benefits of their drug in relation to those of their competitors in their presentation to health-care professionals and are not above manipulating and even rewarding doctors and other health-care professionals with expensive dinners and vacations in order to get them to use their company's products.

A few years ago, it started to dawn on me that many of the drug reps knew precisely how many prescriptions I write monthly for any given drug they represent. Shortly thereafter I learned how they do this: They *buy* the information. It should not come as a surprise that most pharmacies now use a computer network to record what was hitherto confidential information, i.e., prescription data, drug, dosage, physician who prescribed the drug, etc. And in this age, where information is a commodity like any other, this extremely sensitive and private information is of course being sold to the pharmaceutical companies, who in turn distribute it to their sales forces. I've tried to look at these data myself, and for the past two years I've asked approximately thirty different pharmaceutical reps to show me the information they are given about me. While they all admit that they have these secret data on me (and every other doctor they call on), they all told me that they were unable to show me the data on my prescription profile their company had purchased. Many of them spoke to their managers before giving me an answer, and most of them suggested that they could lose their job if they ever showed me my own profile.

Every month the sales rep is given a report on the doctors in his or her territory and how many prescriptions they have written for a specific drug. A field manager then meets with the rep, and together they target those physicians not meeting the goals the company has set for them. Large group practices that prescribe huge quantities of drugs obviously get the most attention. Specialists are besieged by an army of reps—specialty reps, they are called—who have even bigger budgets to spend on the doctor.

The rep then calls on the doctor, often with an offer of a free meal and even an assortment of promotional gifts. During the ensuing discussion the rep usually asks the physician if he prescribes the drug (already knowing, of course, how often the doctor prescribes the drug). If I don't prescribe that particular drug (almost always for a very good reason), I am prepared for any one of several sales-rep tactics. Some ask me, or implore me, even beg me, to please use their drug so they can meet their quota. Others try to manipulate study data to "reeducate" me. The vast majority, however, simply try to coax me with rewards.

How do they do this without breaking the law? There are many tricks in this trade. Very often, the doctor is asked if he would like to go out to dinner with a few other physicians or with his staff in order to discuss a particular medical topic, or, say, the drug in question. This sort of inducement is commonly offered to physicians in private practice, to full-time faculty members in a teaching institution, and to residents in training as well. The rep picks a famous eatery or a nice new place that just got a five-star rating in the local paper. He spends perhaps $1,000 on food and wine for eight or ten physicians engaged in a roundtable discussion. A good time is had by all. Usually, there is a round table, but there is little or no discussion. Pharmaceutical companies have an almost unlimited budget dedicated to "educating" doctors and their staffs in the superior merits of their products. The evening is simply documented on the representative's expense report as "continuing medical education," and it sails cleanly through that loophole in the law.

Physicians who prescribe large quantities of a particular drug, say, an orthopedist who prescribes Vioxx (Merck) and Celebrex (Pfizer), may be treated to sumptuous dinners costing hundreds of dollars per person or enrolled in a seminar (with his or her spouse) valued at thousands of dollars. The assumption being that physicians are going to take a course to learn more about a disease or product. I know an elderly orthopedist with a personal net worth of several million dollars who has often bragged to me about these boondoggles. The seminar is of course a deception created by the company. The lectures are far from mandatory and in any event take no more than a small handful of hours out of a day that is to be spent enjoying the ski slopes or golf links at a five-star resort in Aspen, Vail, Scottsdale, etc.

And if you wish to lecture for the company and get paid perhaps $1,500 for an hour-long talk, you'd better prescribe that drug in large numbers. In 2002, I did some lecturing for a large pharmaceutical company that manufactures a type of drug called a beta-blocker. Yet in spite of a very positive response from the physicians I spoke with (I actually received many consults from these physicians after my talk), I was not asked to continue. When I questioned one of the company's field reps, I received the following reply: "Someone somewhere got the idea that generics are your first choice for the treatment of hypertension and angina." Which of course is the truth. I use the best and least expensive drug (often a generic drug) to treat my patients, but you can clearly see the reason they pay physicians to give talks about a topic.

On January 19, 2003, an Associated Press article titled "Drug Sales Reps Sitting in on Exams" was published. While this appeared as a news story, I can vouch that this practice has been going on since I began my practice, or for at least twelve years. In the article a spokesman for Eli Lilly and Company (manufacturer of drugs like Prozac) acknowledges that reps have been observing doctors treat patients (often patients with very personal problems, such as those seeing psychiatrists) but according to a Lilly spokesman, the doctors must obtain a patient's consent first.[4] The business calls this "shadowing," and I must say that most of my colleagues have been shadowed at one time or another by reps who work for many of the pharmaceutical companies. The drug companies claim they send their reps into doctors' offices to observe and to learn, but frankly, it is just another way for the pharmaceutical companies to "pay off" the doctor (usually $250 to $500) and perhaps (while they are in his office standing over him as he writes his script) intimidate him into writing scripts for their product.

"The AMA does not have policy on shadowing, but one is needed—especially if doctors are being paid," said Dr. Edward Hill, chairman of the AMA Board of Trustees.[5] To Dr. Hill I say, "Where have you been for the past ten-plus years?"

The doctor of course is frequently a more-than-willing co-conspirator in these ventures, and sometimes more corrupt than the corporation so assiduously trying to get him to prescribe its drugs. Over the past few years I have inquired of many a pharmaceutical rep just what is going on in the medical community of which I am a member. I've been told that there are doctors who have asked them for money for donations to a society of doctors of which they are a part, for lavish dinner parties for family and friends, for golf outings, trips around the world (which as I mentioned earlier are done under the ruse of a medical conference), and, perhaps worst of all, for drug samples in large volumes, which the doctor then sells illegally for huge financial gains.

And if you don't believe me, just read part of a statement released in April 2003 from the Office of Inspector General (OIG):

> Drug companies are further cautioned about physician marketing activities, including making excessive payments for physician's consulting and research services, and offering inappropriate entertainment, recreation, travel, meals, gifts, gratuities, and other business courtesies to physicians and other health care providers who influence the prescribing of drugs. Payments by drug companies to physicians and pharmacists to switch patients to their drugs from a competitor's are cited as problematic, as are payments to a physician to listen to a drug representative's sales presentation.[6]

Another part of that statement speaks of the improper and illegal sale of sample medications: "These sales have emerged as a major risk because of violations revealed by recent enforcement activities and the widespread industry practice of providing free samples to physicians." The OIG further states that "both the antikickback statute and the False Claims Act may be implicated when the federal health care programs are billed for samples in violation of the Prescription Drug Marketing Act of 1987."[7]

Perhaps the most common question from the admittedly less brazen but no less on-the-make physician is: "What will you do for me if I start prescribing your medication?" I have a suspicion that few if any of the reps who read this book will deny that they have been propositioned in some way by a physician.

The bottom line here, unfortunately, is that many physicians have been allowed, even encouraged, to consider their own best interests, as well as those of the pharmaceutical industry and its shareholders, at precisely the moment when their sole priority should be the health and well-being of their patients. Consider the physician, for example, who yields to one or more of the techniques illustrated above and prescribes a $6/day drug such as Coreg for high blood pressure (50 mg of Coreg twice daily) when he might have chosen an equally efficacious medication from the same drug class, such as atenolol, which costs as little as eleven cents a day (based on the highest recommended dose and price at Drugstore.com). Here, I suppose, if you are lucky, only your wallet, as well as that of your insurance company, is effected by the industry's powers of persuasion.

But let's ponder what can happen when your physician yields to pressure and selects a drug that is *not* as helpful to you as the less-expensive alternative. There are uncounted physicians out there right now who are in many cases foolishly prescribing any one of several of the most overprescribed class of drugs right now, namely the calcium channel blockers (CCBs), which are approved for use in cases of hypertension, angina, and coronary disease in general. (Norvasc, to use just one example, grossed over $4.3 billion for Pfizer in 2002.)[8] Do you have to wonder any longer why drugs like Norvasc, or Cardizem, or Tiazac, or Procardia, or Adalat, or Cardene, or DynaCirc are so often prescribed by doctors, generating billions of dollars in revenue for the huge pharmaceutical companies like Pfizer, Forrest Labs, Biovail, Roche Laboratories, and Novartis, when there is *no evidence* that they improve survival rates in cases of coronary heart disease, angina, or heart failure? (Some studies suggest that some of these drugs might even *increase* mortality in patients with heart failure, an acute heart attack, or unstable angina when compared with a placebo!) More pressure tactics from the big pharmaceutical companies, to be sure.

Let's say, for example, that you are a diabetic and your doctor prescribes one of these calcium channel blockers for your hypertension, but neglects to also prescribe another type of drug called an angiotensin converting enzyme inhibitor (ACEI). Sadly, you are receiving inappropriate care. No drug other than one from the class of drugs called ACEI or receptor blockers (ARBs) should ever be prescribed to a diabetic patient with high blood pressure (unless there is a reason the patient cannot take that drug, or additional drugs are needed to lower the patient's blood pressure).

So why, several times a week, week in and week out, do I see diabetic patients who are being treated by other physicians with only a CCB for their high blood pressure? And why were patients by the thousands being prescribed drugs like Baycol (which has caused deaths due to mysositis) or Posicor (which has caused deaths due to arrhythmias and dangerous interactions with other medications), when there have been other thoroughly tested and safe drugs on the market for years that we physicians all knew were at least equally efficacious? I think you know why now.

Here is some very clear and categorical advice: Never under any circumstances accept a new drug (which I would define as a drug that has been on the market for less than one year) if there are similar drugs that have been on the market—and thus prescribed to perhaps a million patients—for years. Drugs like Baycol, Posicor, and Rezulin were shown to be safe in rather large patient studies, yet like the infamous Thalidamide, were found to be quite dangerous only after a larger patient population took the drug. Think about it. It just makes sense that adverse or even deadly effects of drugs might not show up in trials, especially if the risk is relatively small.

Let's say it turns out that in practice drug A causes deadly liver damage in 0.01 percent (one hundredth of one percent) of patients. It is highly likely, then, in a study conducted on as many as 5,000 patients, that this deadly adverse effect would not be revealed. Yet when the drug is released to market and perhaps 1 million patients are prescribed this drug, then as many as 100 people would probably be killed by a drug whose safety is based on a good scientific study.

And even if the drug is safe when taken by itself, once it is available in the general community and prescribed to patients already on other prescription drugs, the combination of this new drug with others could form a deadly cocktail in the blood, just as Posicor and Seldane did. Both medications, when combined with other prescription drugs, or even with low levels of blood potassium, caused deadly arrhythmias. Posicor, for example, was approved in 1997 by the FDA but removed from the market in 1998 after causing at least 143 deaths. I've never prescribed this drug because I knew that we have had similar drugs on the market for years. Yet how well I remember the expensive dinners and the top-quality stethoscopes the drug manufacturer offered to physicians in its efforts to get them to prescribe the drug to their patients.

What is particularly bothersome, and quite frankly stupid, is that our FDA uses the same panel of physicians who approved the drug to make the decision to pull the drug off the market. Thus, the panel has to come to grips with the fact that they made a bad decision, admit their error, and then reverse their previous decision. Countries like the United Kingdom have separate expert panels of physicians who make the decision to withdraw a drug from the market. Perhaps that is why Rezulin, which was approved by the FDA in January 1997, was finally taken off the market (and voluntarily by its manufacturer) fully three years later, in 2000.

For the past twenty years, a physician named Dr. Marvin Moser has tirelessly and courageously advocated the use of an inexpensive water pill as the first choice for patients with high blood pressure. And for the past twenty years many physicians have ridiculed him for doing so. Yet, we now know beyond a shadow of a doubt that he was right all along.

On December 17, 2002, the results of a landmark study conducted by the National Heart, Lung and Blood Institute (NHLBI)—an agency of our government—were published in the *Journal of the American Medical Association* (*JAMA*). Called the ALLHAT (Antihypertensive and Lipid-Lowering Treatment to Prevent Heart Attack Trial), it was conducted over the course of eight years and studied 42,418 high-risk hypertensive patients. Patients were randomly given one of four drugs: a water pill (chlorthalidone), a calcium channel blocker (amlodipine/Norvasc), an angiotensin-converting enzyme inhibitor (lisinopril); or an alpha-blocker (doxazosin/Cardura). In March 2000, however, the doxazocin arm of the study was stopped because too many patients taking that medication (when compared with those on the water pill) were developing heart failure. Therefore, at the completion of the study, there were only three drugs whose effects were still being studied. Remarkably, the least expensive drug—the water pill—was found to be the most effective.[9] Chlorthalidone, a drug you can purchase for less than 10¢ a pill, was found to be more effective in preventing the onset of heart failure than Pfizer's Norvasc, which costs over $1.50/day for a comparable dose.

The authors of the trial concluded: "The results of ALLHAT indicate that thiazide-type diuretics should be considered first for pharmacologic therapy in patients with hypertension. They are unsurpassed in lowering BP, reducing clinical events, and tolerability, and they are less costly."[10]

Does it come as any surprise that of all the huge studies conducted and paid for by the pharmaceutical industry, not one study compared an expensive brand-name drug with the pennies-per-day water pill, chlorthalidone? Why? As Deep Throat said over and over to Bob Woodward and Carl Bernstein, like a mantra, *follow the money*. In 2002, Pfizer realized sales of Norvasc totaling $4.3 billion! Let me put it another way. A three-months' supply of a 10-mg dose of Norvasc (the highest dose of this drug given in the NHLBI study) costs $167.37 at Drugstore.com. The same three-month's supply of the 25-mg dose of the water pill (the highest dose given in the study) can be purchased for a mere $8.78 at the same online site. If you were a Pfizer executive, would you have been pleased to see—and been willing to publicize—the results of the NHLBI study? Hardly.

Will Pfizer sell $4.3 billion worth of Norvasc in 2003 given the incontrovertible results of the NHLBI study? I suspect not; they'll probably sell even more. How can this be?

Because the pharmaceutical companies are very clever, cunning, and devious in their tactics. First, they might attempt to ignore the ALLHAT study (as they do with any study that might show a particular drug to be better than theirs). As big and important as this trial was, the huge pharmaceuticals, like Pfizer, hope that with time and lack of media coverage the memories of this landmark trial will fade. If the results had gone the other way and the trial had showed definitively that an expensive drug made by company X was better than the others, then company X would have had billboards made up and purchased radio and TV time on the Super Bowl telling you about it. Ah, but the results concluded that an 8¢/day medication is better than the $1.50/day med, and that drug (with its small margin of profit) is manufactured by companies that don't have billion-dollar marketing teams. So the "we'll pay no attention to it and they'll forget about it" policy is, I suspect, the first step.

If that step is unsuccessful (and it may not be if enough people read this book), then the huge pharmaceuticals will attack.

Perhaps they will go after me by paying high-profile experts in the field of hypertension to attack what I have written or to attack the results of the trial. They'll focus on the adverse effects of the water pill, which include possible insulin resistance (thus increasing sugars in susceptible patients), elevated lipids (although most believe this is a transient effect), and the risk of gout. They'll find something in the ALLHAT results that was favorable to their drug and promote that result. These arguments will have some thread of truth, but they will be unable to confront the primary result of the trial that patients (even if they had diabetes, smoked, or had high cholesterol) on the 8¢/day water pill maintained better health.

They may attempt to frighten physicians by conjuring up future potential risks of this water pill. For example, five years ago I sat through a cardiology lecture at our institution given by a very famous cardiologist who told us (based on small anecdotal reports) that water pills could cause kidney cancer and told us we would be reading about this in the medical journals in a few years. I'm still waiting.

The huge pharmaceuticals might sponsor seminars for physicians to attend (in five-star hotels) or increase their marketing budgets so they can take doctors to dinner or golf outings. They'll flood the physicians' offices with free samples of their drugs so the physician can save the patient a trip to the pharmacy—to get the $3/day drug. And finally, and this is my personal experience, reps will plead with the physicians to use their drug because their salaried bonus depends on their sales.

I just hope they don't attack me in the same manner that they attacked Dr. Moser or Dr. Susan Love. Dr. Love is another physician who was unjustly ridiculed by the medical establishment for years. Until 2002 anyway.

In 1997, a study published in the *New England Journal of Medicine* (*NEJM*) noted a significant reduction in mortality in postmenopausal women who took the hormone estrogen. In addition, the study concluded that women who took estrogen had a 53 percent reduction in mortality due to heart disease. The final sentence of the article stated, crucially, "On average, the survival benefits appear to outweigh the risks, but the risks and benefits vary depending on existing risk factors and the duration of hormone use and must be carefully considered for each woman."[11]

As soon as the study was published, American Home Products (now known as Wyeth) was off to the races, promoting their estrogen drug, Premarin. Many physicians, including me, sat through lectures (sometimes sponsored by AHP) designed to promote the use of estrogen in postmenopausal women. Sure enough, sales of Premarin soon went through the roof (over $1.3 billion in 1997 alone), even though many if not most physicians had serious doubts about the validity of the type of study that showed these apparent health benefits.

This study, called a case-control study, compared women who were taking the drug with those who were not. But it was based on a questionnaire filled out by nurses, and even more important, it was not a classic, well-controlled double-blind randomized study. (Again, the latter is a study in which half the women would have been given a placebo pill and the other half the estrogen pill with neither the doctor nor the patients knowing which pill they were taking.) Moreover, the results of this case-control study could very easily be skewed and/or just plain wrong.

For example, what if for some reason fit, diet-conscious women took estrogen while unfit women did not? We know that fit and diet-conscious people are less likely to have heart attacks. At the time, however, there was no shortage of experts who insisted that the study results were most probably true. Many of these "experts," however, had some sort of financial relationship with American Home Products, the maker of Premarin.

Dr. Susan Love, then the director of the Revlon/UCLA Breast Center, was one of the few unbiased experts who remained consistently skeptical of these study results. In her book, *Dr. Susan Love's Hormone Book,* she rejected the widespread advocacy of estrogen hormone replacement for elderly women. Dr. Love worried about the increased risk of breast cancer in these women as well as the risk of blood clots. She also pointed out that there was bias in the selection process employed by the *NEJM* study. In particular, she wrote, "The women who took estrogen were of higher socioeconomic status, better educated, thinner and more likely to be non-smokers."[12] She concluded that these women were "therefore more likely to have had overall preventive care, such as having their blood pressure checked and their cholesterol monitored."[13] This was precisely the sort of flawed study design that so many of us had been worried about initially but which had been so vigorously defended by the "experts."

Dr. Love's excellent observations and her attack on this widespread abuse of estrogen therapy made her a favorite target of most of the scientific community. Pharmaceutical reps I met loved nothing more than to ridicule her theories. At a meeting of the American College of Obstetrics and Gynecology (ACOG), one doctor who attended a debate between Dr. Love and a senior member of that society later wrote, "never in my experience have I witnessed a more biased, personalized, and condescending attack on a fellow physician than the public attack made by the president of ACOG on Dr. Love." Doctor Love wrote to me to add that she had a couple of speaking engagements canceled and one where she was told that she could talk about breast cancer but not HRT (hormone replacement therapy)—she of course turned down that speaking engagement. The fact is, most of us (including me, at first) were convinced—by the experts—that not only was she wrong, but that her well-publicized opinions were causing the deaths of thousands of women.

In 1997, *The New Yorker* published an essay by Malcolm Gladwell (who to my knowledge has no affiliation with the pharmaceutical industry) called "The Estrogen Question: How Wrong Is Dr. Susan Love?" (You can read the entire article at *http://www.gladwell.com/1997/1997_06_09_a_estrogen.htm.*) Mr. Gladwell portrays Dr. Love as someone who is out of touch with reality. In his lengthy and one-sided portrayal of the doctor he writes: "So why, after even the slightest scrutiny, does so much of what Love has to say begin to fall apart?" He also states that "hormone replacement therapy lowers the risk of heart disease by somewhere between forty and fifty percent . . ."[14] How wrong is Mr. Gladwell? Read on and you shall see.

In 1998, the Heart and Estrogen Progestin Replacement Study (HERS) published by the *Journal of the American Medical Association* showed that HRT did not reduce the risk of heart attack or death from heart disease in postmenopausal women with known heart disease. It also noted that in spite of the favorable effect HRT had on cholesterol, in the first year of the study more women who took the drug had heart attacks than those who did not.[15] At that point I began advising all my patients to stop taking HRT, and I have not prescribed it since.

Amazingly, the advocates of HRT set out to spin the study results. Since this was a study on women who already had heart disease, they asked, how do we know that HRT doesn't help the millions of women without heart disease who take the drug to prevent heart attack and stroke? Once again, the market wizards and the doctors who worked for Wyeth managed to keep the sales of Premarin over $1.4 billion that year.

In 2003, the Women's Health Initiative study was terminated early because it showed that in the women who took HRT (in this case, a combination of estrogen and progestin), the risk of coronary artery disease, breast cancer, stroke, and lung clots was increased![16] Dr. Love was right! The theory and selling pitch that hormone replacement therapy was a safe and effective way to reduce death in postmenopausal women was wrong. End of story, right?

After the publication of the WHI study, an article commenting on its effect appeared in *Business Week* on September 16, 2002, as well as another smaller study on sales of HRT by Wyeth.

S&P [Standard & Poor's] believes that the cancer risks in the NCI study were generally known for years, and the absolute incidence of adverse events in both studies were extremely small. For example, the risk of breast cancer in the WHI study was only 8 women in 10,000. In addition, the adverse events appeared mainly after five years of use, while most women typically are on HRT therapy for shorter periods.

Although the number of HRT prescriptions written dropped sharply in the first few weeks after the news, more recent data showed that weekly figures stabilized and began to inch up. While fallout from the studies and a more restrictive label are likely to result in a 15% drop in Premarin/Prempro sales in 2002, Wyeth's total HRT sales should stabilize at about $1.4 billion annual rate over the next few years.[17]

Recently, thank goodness, the FDA announced that it is requiring Wyeth and all other companies making drugs that contain estrogen with or without progestin to carry a black box warning, the highest level of caution in warning label information. In addition to noting the increased risk for heart attacks, strokes, blood clots, and breast cancer, the warning also stresses that these products are not approved for preventing heart disease.[18]

But just the other day, I read an article in a medical journal about HRT in postmenopausal women. In it, the author suggested that there are still many potential uses for HRT in postmenopausal women. She also acknowledged that she has received research support from Wyeth Pharmaceuticals.

But even more discouraging was what a patient told me as I was writing this chapter. I consulted on a postmenopausal woman who was given HRT by her gynecologist for some dryness only a year ago. She had a very strong family history of coronary disease and thus was sent to me. I told her about the risks of taking the hormones and asked if her doctor had explained them to her. Her reply was "No. He handed me a prescription and told me it would make me feel better."

There is a lesson to be learned from this. First, always ask your doctor about the risks of taking medications. Second, fire any doctor who with some sort of thoughtless gesture tells you to take a medication because it will make you feel better. Finally, go home and read about what you are taking, and if you are unsure, call your doctor up or go see another physician for a second opinion. I cannot stress how important it is to get a second opinion on any topic that you feel unsure about.

This entire HRT episode, it seems to me, is a tale of two tragedies. First, as you have seen, going against the behemoth that is big medicine, for any reason, all too often brings swift, unrelenting, and devastating ridicule and denunciation down upon the head of the individual with enough courage and integrity to challenge its authority. Dr. Love should have been singled out for praise and commendations when she tried to convince the public and her fellow physicians that HRT was far from a panacea, *especially after several studies proved her correct.* Yet you can see how she was treated for her gallant efforts. Even when she was proven right, she still did not receive public apologies.

Second, in spite of the incontestable results of all the published data, Wyeth continues to bring in well over $1 billion in HRT sales annually. And there is even more. On June 9, 2003, the FDA approved a new, lower-dose version of Prempro. The approval of this drug was accompanied by a statement by Wyeth vice president Victoria Kusiak: "These approvals mean that women and clinicians will have two low-dose options to better individualize effective treatment for menopausal symptom relief and concomitant bone protection."[19] In other words, Wyeth has come out with lower doses of the drug that they can say were not studied (i.e., condemned) in the huge trials I just described. Thus, they can market their drug again and cynically, and perhaps dangerously (if the lower dose of therapy also increases the possibility of bad events) placate the public's justified fear about the dangers of HRT. And I wonder—since it takes several years and millions of dollars to conduct a study that would be needed to show any benefit or risk of the low-dose drug—if a study will ever be done. And if one is in fact initiated, you can be sure that billions of dollars worth of the drug will have already been sold to women before the results are in. What a sad commentary on the mind-set and manipulative schemes of the entire drug industry.

A second front in the pharmaceutical companies' efforts to corner the market for a particular drug is the hospital. There, special hospital reps (usually with more senior positions at the company) call on the pharmacists, faculty attending physicians, and the residents in training, but the same scenario occurs, with trips and expensive dinners given out to any person who might be in a position to influence a more aggressive use of the reps' drugs. Again, most of these big-ticket items end up on an expense report filled out by the rep under a heading for continuing education (for example, "residents and attending doctors attending discussion on drug X at restaurant A").

But there are other ways to skin a cat. With limited budgets and inventory space, most in-hospital pharmacies are forced to limit the number of drugs they have *on formulary*—that is, drugs they actually stock. For example, there are now six statin drugs available for lowering cholesterol. Most hospitals stock only one and will automatically substitute the agent they have in stock for any others that might be prescribed.

This is a classic example of how pharmaceutical companies, in this case Merck, will work with local hospitals to try to dominate the market at the expense of the patient.

On April 20, 1998, in order to prevent a further decline in the sales (compared to those of the relative newcomer Lipitor, from Pfizer) of their blockbuster cholesterol-lowering drug Zocor (one of the most expensive drugs in its class), Merck created a program to encourage hospitals all across the country to use their drug instead of any one of a small handful of other equally effective medications. Here is how one of the most scandalous schemes I have ever encountered during my career in medicine works. Merck sells the drug to hospitals at a 92 percent discount (rather than the usual discount of 10 or at most 25 percent) as long as it is dispensed more than 70 percent of the time for that type of drug (called statins). Hospitals are only too eager to keep their costs down, and thus they comply with Merck's budgetary persuasion by placing Zocor as the only statin drug on the hospital formulary.

Essentially, this means that Zocor is automatically supplied to a patient when the pharmacy receives a prescription for any other drug in that drug class. The doctor must fill out a lengthy form if he wants to insist that another drug be administered. Overnight, Zocor gained the ability to develop a huge market share over the other statins. You may know them as Lipitor, Crestor, Pravachol, Lescol, Mevacor, and Baycol. (After causing over 100 deaths Baycol was taken off the market.) Merck, of course, hopes that the patient will be discharged on Zocor, since he or she was receiving the medicine in the hospital. And this is very often what happens in hospitals where overworked residents and house doctors just prescribe the medication listed on the patient's chart when they are ready to go home. These house doctors are not familiar with the patient and won't be seeing him or her again. So in situations like this the patient may receive a prescription whether or not it is precisely the best medication for that patient's specific health issues.

In fact, this very thing recently happened to my father. My dad went to Beth Israel Hospital in New York City on Lipitor but left with prescriptions from the house doctors for both Coumadin, which he needed to take to prevent a blood clot in his leg, and Zocor, the only available statin in that hospital. Only with very careful monitoring of his Coumadin level (called an INR) were we able to place him back on his Lipitor, of which he already had a three-month supply at home. I'm sure other patients (whose sons are not physicians) would either go out and buy the new drug, even though they might have months' worth of the other statin at home, or substitute one drug for the other, unaware of the risky interaction one might have with a blood thinner like Coumadin.

At the university hospital where I am a clinical professor of medicine, Zocor is automatically substituted for whatever statin drug a newly admitted patient has been taking outside. However, it is well known that Zocor can interact dangerously with several medications that similar drugs, like Lipitor, Pravachol, and Lescol, may not. In fact, even Merck, the manufacturer of Zocor, recently published warnings about the use of their drug with several other drugs, including blood pressure medications like verapamil, certain medications used for HIV patients, certain antibiotics like erythromycin and Biaxin, and even large quantities of grapefruit juice (over a quart per day).[20] Did you know that?

When I receive a request for a prescription change (from Lipitor to Zocor) from the Merck-Medco Rx Services, the following advisory is included: "Patients on warfarin are excluded because a change to Zocor may affect the INR." This means that patients taking the blood thinner Coumadin (warfarin) and Zocor can develop dangerous bleeds because Zocor can increase the effectiveness of Coumadin. This warning is not given on the computer system we use, and when I randomly polled 20 doctors about the matter, only one knew about this adverse effect. Essentially, in every hospital where I am an attending physician, patients taking warfarin and Lipitor, Pravachol, or any of the other statins are having their statin changed to Zocor. Coumadin bleeding levels (a measurement used to see how the blood's ability to clot is affected—called an INR) are thus being adversely affected and some patients may have life-threatening bleeds in the hospital (while on Zocor), or strokes when they leave the hospital and resume taking their other statin. Merck has had to notify doctors in writing about this matter, essentially agreeing with what I am saying.

The other truly reprehensible part of this scheme by Merck involves the expense for the patient. Zocor is a more costly drug for the patient. At Montefiore Medical Center in the Bronx, New

York, patients (many of whom are strapped financially) are being discharged and converted to Zocor by physicians who are unaware of what a duplicitous plan they are taking part in.

In my random sample of three pharmacies located near the hospital, a starting dose of 20 mg of Zocor ranged from a low of $128.95 to a high of $142, with the midmost being $135, while its strongest competitor, Lipitor (10 mg), from Pfizer, was priced at $69, $66.95, and $69, respectively. The table on page 194 shows the Average Wholesale Pricing (AWP) for the different statin drugs. This is based on data taken from a standard source called the *Red Book*—in this case, from the April 2003 issue—that pharmacies throughout the country use to determine the price of a drug.[21]

As you can see, while Merck sells Zocor for pennies a pill to the hospital, Zocor remains one of the most expensive statins for a patient to purchase from the hospital. Once out of the hospital, the patient or his insurance company must pay perhaps twice as much money as he or they would for an equally effective drug. I spoke with several Merck reps about this, and they acknowledged that Zocor is more expensive than most of the other statins available. Each one, however, had the same excuse: "If the patient has a drug plan, then their insurance will pick up the expense anyway."

Statins are medications that are very often taken for life. Thus, those patients who have been switched to Zocor might pay as much as an additional $24,000 over a twenty-year period ($1,200 per year). All because of a scheme carried out by Merck with the collaboration of many of the best-known hospitals throughout the United States.

Drugs	FDA-Approved Daily Dosage	Usual Decrease in LDL Cholesterol	Average Wholesale Price, in $
Lipitor (Pfizer)	Initial: 10 mg once Maximum: 80 mg once	35%–40% 50%–60%	214.70/90 tabs. 327.93/90 tabs.
*Baycol (Bayer)			
Lescol (Novartis)	Initial: 20 mg once Maximum: 40 mg bid	20%–25% 30%–35%	177.88/100 tabs. 177.88/100 tabs.
Mevacor (Merck)	Initial: 20 mg once Maximum: 80 mg (two 40-mg tabs.) once	25%–30% 35%–40%	268.39/100 tabs. 247.80/100 tabs.
Pravachol (Bristol-Myers Squibb)	Initial: 20 mg once Maximum: 80 mg once	25%–32% 30%–37%	277.24/90 tabs. 406.84/90 tabs.
Zocor (Merck)	Initial: 20 mg once Maximum: 80 mg once	35%–40% 45%–50%	416.66/90 tabs. 412.66/90 tabs.

*In 2001, Baycol was removed from the market due to deaths caused by myositis.

Source of wholesale prices: *Red Book: Drug Topics*. Thompson Micromedex (Montvale, NJ, April 2003).

Here's still another example of the kinds of tactics that are used by pharmaceutical companies. Since the 1980s cardiologists have used a potent intravenous drug called heparin to prevent heart attacks in patients with a syndrome called unstable angina. In the late 1990s, a new class of similar drugs, called low-molecular-weight heparin (LMWH), were developed and studied, and one, called Lovenox (Aventis), was found to reduce heart attacks and recurrent chest pain in more patients than the first heparin.[22]

Sure enough, a still newer version of this LMWH, called Fragmin (Pharmacia), was subsequently tested in a smaller study (with fewer patients). It was shown to be only as effective as the traditional Heparin (FRIC Trial Circulation, July 1997),[23] yet hundreds of hospitals throughout the United States are now closing their formulary to Lovenox (meaning you cannot get the drug in these hospitals) in favor of Fragmin because the drug's manufacturer has provided the hospitals with huge discounts, just as Merck did with Zocor.

At Montefiore Medical Center in New York City, the annual savings of converting all LMWH to Fragmin was estimated to be $250,000. In July 2000, a task force that included doctors and senior pharmacists decided after researching both drugs that Lovenox and Fragmin were therapeutic equivalents and gave the go-ahead for Fragmin to be the exclusive LMWH available at the hospital. Of interest, one of the senior pharmacists on that task force later left Montefiore to work for Pharmacia, the makers of Fragmin. This information (save for the part about the pharmacist's new job) was provided under section 2805-M of the public health law and is in response to the quality assurance coordinating council.

But that's not all, folks. In the 1990s, Merck acquired Medco Containment Inc., a large wholesale drug distributor, now called Merck-Medco Rx Services, that contracts directly with many of the largest HMOs to supply their patient's medications. Would it surprise you to learn that shortly after that merger, I began to receive multiple letters and faxes every day from Merck or Merck-Medco, urging me to exchange one medication (someone else's) for another similar one (theirs) because the one I prescribed was not on formulary at a given HMO? Here is an example of one of these letters:

> Your patient's prescription benefit plan has adopted a formulary as part of its overall cost containment objectives. Please determine the preferred medication listed in this request is appropriate for this patient and respond accordingly. This change does not determine benefit coverage. As with any change in drug therapy, please consider the individual drug product characteristics and individual patient factors such as: coexisting disease states, contraindications, therapeutic history, present medications, and other relevant circumstances.

Essentially, though, the company keeps harassing the doctor until he or she responds or changes the patient's medication. Most physicians just change the medication, in this case from Lipitor to Zocor. And of course, as you know by now, Merck manufactures Zocor.

One final note on Merck and Medco Health Solutions. In August of 2003, Merck spun off Medco as a separate company. It is now being traded on the NYSE as a separate corporate entity.

While we are on the subject of Merck's propensity for manipulating markets, hospitals, and HMOs, it is worth noting the presence of one other drug on my comparison chart above, namely Mevacor, since it is the oldest and perhaps least-effective drug in lowering cholesterol. Compared to Lipitor 10 mg, which costs $61.99 at Drugstore.com (price as of June 2003), the cost of an equivalent amount of Mevacor 80 mg is $246 at the same pharmacy. So, why would an older drug with more side effects, drug interactions, and the inconvenience of night dosing (instead of anytime in the day for Lipitor) cost over four times as much as the best-selling statin?

Well, for one thing, Mevacor became available in generic form in 2002. A generic drug is a drug that no longer is patented by a specific pharmaceutical company. This usually occurs ten years after the company is first granted approval for its use by the FDA. When a drug becomes generic it can be produced with FDA approval by several other pharmaceutical companies, and thus the price of the drug is usually substantially reduced, sometimes to as little as a mere 5 percent of the cost of the patented drug.

Of note, Mevacor is now known as Lovastatin in its generic form, and is priced at $62.99 for a 40-mg dosage instead of $122.99 for the brand name. Frankly, at over $2 a pill, the generic version is no bargain.[24] I wonder why it costs so much. In my eperience, if you cut your pill of 10 mg of Lipitor in half, you have equal efficacy at a price even lower than that of the generic. Plus don't forget to ask your doctor for samples. Pfizer delivers them to your doctor by the case.

In my view Merck has artificially raised the price of Mevacor because it wishes to use a little financial arm-twisting to encourage the patients who have been faithfully and happily taking Mevacor to switch to Zocor, which is still protected by their patents. By keeping the price of Mevacor relatively high they are able to extract every last dollar of profit they can before it is available as a generic and at the same time make their Zocor look like a relative bargain to those loyal patients who have taken Mevacor for years but who now feel compelled, financially, to switch. The individuals determined to stay with the brand Mevacor will have to continue to pay these high prices unless they switch to the generic.

It shouldn't surprise you to know that the large pharmaceutical companies are against FDA approval of any generic substitutes of their drug since they are in a position to lose billions of dollars as a result. And even after the generic versions do become readily available, many of these companies have their reps visit doctors' offices to suggest to the doctors that they should write "Dispense as Written (DAW)" on the name-brand drug. DAW tells the pharmacist that he cannot substitute an almost exact generic duplicate of the drug. For years, the companies have even suggested—*insinuated* is a better word—that a generic drug is simply not as good as its patented counterpart, despite careful FDA scrutiny and no hard evidence to support this claim.

Here is a case in point. Coumadin is the brand-name drug of warfarin, a potent blood thinner used to prevent stroke and other forms of clots. It's a very effective drug, and there's no question that Coumadin/warfarin has saved countless lives since it was introduced well over forty years ago.

During my residency and well into my private practice sales reps from DuPont brought samples of Coumadin to the clinics and office and always reminded us that the brand Coumadin was much safer and purer than the generic drug; it was also much more expensive. Unlike most drugs on the market the effects of Coumadin/warfarin need to be monitored at least every month. Too much of it, and you might hemorrhage; too little, and the drug doesn't work. Levels of the clotting factors (which the drug affects) can be altered significantly by even a change in diet or, as we were led to believe, by inferior generic copies of Coumadin, since they might not be absorbed as well or perhaps differ in dosage from tablet to tablet. Because many of us believed what the DuPont reps said, we were frightened to prescribe the generic warfarin. Until recently that is.

In 2001 DuPont, the manufacturer of Coumadin, settled class-action lawsuits for $44.5 million in the U.S. District Court of Delaware. Under the terms of the proposed settlement, the defendant DuPont agreed to establish a settlement fund in the amount of $44.5 million, plus interest, although it denied all wrongdoing in this case. In these cases plaintiffs alleged that DuPont violated the law by, among other things, disseminating false and misleading information, claiming that there is a lack of "bioequivalence or therapeutic equivalence between Coumadin and other warfarin sodium products, and by providing consideration to entities involved in the distribution of pharmaceuticals to induce them to favor Coumadin over other warfarin sodium products, which allegations DuPont denies."[25]

DuPont sold its rights to Coumadin to Bristol-Myers Squibb last year. Recently a rep from Bristol came to my office in an attempt to market the drug. He shouted to me, "Hey doc, I hope you're not using generic warfarin. You know the levels of the generics are all over the place." So, I asked him if Bristol ever told him about the lawsuit DuPont settled because of statements like that. He chuckled and said no. By the way, the price of the average dose of Coumadin (5 mg) is $61.99 for a ninety-day supply at Drugstore.com, while the same supply of 5-mg tablets of warfarin is $34.99.

The well-known fact that many large pharmaceutical companies often manufacture their own generic version of their brand-name drug at the same plant, but on alternate days, should tell you all you need to know about the arrogance and hypocrisy of these firms.

I have to confess that I can only laugh, with a very dark sense of humor, indeed, at the drug companies who stop pushing a drug or advertising it on television just before the patent for that drug expires and a new, generic equivalent becomes available. Turn on your television and there is Nexium being hailed as the latest panacea for ulcers and heartburn. Last year, Prilosec was the drug to take. Both of these drugs, by the way, are manufactured by the drug giant, AstraZeneca Pharmaceuticals. And while AstraZeneca has conducted clinical trials showing some improved healing, in reality, none of the physicians I spoke with believe that in the clinical setting Nexium is truly superior to Prilosec.

What they will tell you is that AstraZeneca is soon expecting to lose at least 50 percent of its market for Prilosec when the new, less-expensive generics become available. Thus, in order to maintain their bottom line for the ladies and gentlemen on Wall Street, they have come up with Nexium, a similar drug with similar activity that is every bit as expensive as Prilosec, if not more so. And even better, it is protected by a new patent. Nexium, of course, is launched in plenty of time to convince all of us to switch to the newer and *better* but more expensive drug.

The hundreds of bottles of samples I once had in my office for Prilosec are all gone, replaced by Nexium. When I ask the reps why they are so generous with their samples, they tell me they are "to help the indigent, to make it easier for the patient who cannot run to the pharmacy that day." So I ask, "Where is all the Prilosec?"

I need to make another point here while we are on the subject of Prilosec. The companies that manufacture generic drugs are not averse to making huge profits (that perhaps even exceed those of the regular pharms, since they didn't spend tens of millions on the research) on a medication, in this case generic Prilosec (omeprazole). Schwarz Pharmaceutical, a German pharmaceutical company, is so far the only company that has been given permission by our FDA to sell omeprazole in the United States. The price of a 20-mg pill remains at $3.33, compared to the brand-name price of $3.86.[26] What's even more troublesome is that our German friends charge only $1.45 for the same generic pill in Germany (source: direct communication with a pharmacist in Germany). All of this became moot in late 2003 when the drug Prilosec went "over the counter."

While I am on this point, I want to express my concern in a more general way about the higher prices U.S. citizens are frequently asked to pay for their drugs by U.S. companies when compared to the prices European firms charge their EU customers. The American firms argue that if they had to charge us similarly discounted prices they wouldn't be able to spend sufficient money for research and development, and perhaps they wouldn't even be able to survive. I guess thanks to powerful lobbyists and our own nationalist spirit, we've put up with these extra charges.

But I was perplexed and upset to find that we pay a huge premium for drugs developed outside our country as well. Take the case of Plavix, a stronger-than-aspirin blood thinner. Ask Jean-Francois Dehecq, chairman and CEO of Sanofi, a French pharmaceutical company, about the sales of Plavix, and he'll tell you that sales are great. Developed by Sanofi but also licensed to and sold by Bristol-Myers Squibb in the United States, sales of Plavix are now well over $1 billion annually.

I found the price of Plavix to be about $108 at Drugstore.com, but under $70 for a month's supply at almost every Canadian pharmacist on the Internet.[27] So why do we spend 50 percent more here for the same pill made by a French company? In early 2003, with talk of war in Iraq the dominant news item, together with France's unwillingness to support the U.S./British–led coalition, I'm quite sure it's not because we're all Francophiles. We could easily lower the cost of medications like Plavix by demanding that drugs developed and manufactured outside the United States (in this case, France) be sold here at the same price as they are sold in Europe.

Below is a list of other popular prescription drugs which are sold by foreign-owned companies in the United States. Some of these drugs are marketed by U. S. companies and therefore many of you probably think they were developed by a U. S. company. One of the most popular prescription drugs is the antihistamine Zyrtec. In July 2003, I e-mailed investor relations at UCB to ask what the average cost of the drug Zyrtec was (an

Drugs Sold in the United States by International Corporations

Prescribed Drugs	Company	Use	Pharmaceutical Headquarters— Country
1. Diovan (valsartan)	Novartis	Hypertension	Basel, Switzerland
2. Neoral (cyclosporine)	Novartis	Immuno-suppressant	Basel, Switzerland
3. Lamisil (terbinafine)	Novartis	Fungal infection	Basel, Switzerland
4. Gleevec (imatinib)	Novartis	Chronic myeloid leukemia (CML)	Basel, Switzerland
5. Atacand (candesartan)	AstraZeneca LP	Hypertension	United Kingdom/ Sweden
6. Casodex (bicalutamide)	AstraZeneca LP	Benign Prostatic Hypertrophy	United Kingdom/ Sweden
7. Nexium (esomeprazole)	AstraZeneca LP	GERD	United Kingdom/ Sweden
8. Prilosec (omeprazole)	AstraZeneca LP	GERD	United Kingdom/ Sweden
9. Toprol XL (metoprolol)	AstraZeneca LP	Hypertension	United Kingdom/ Sweden
10. Zoladex (goserelin)	AstraZeneca LP	Prostatic cancer, endometriosis, or breast cancer	United Kingdom/ Sweden

Prescribed Drugs	Company	Use	Pharmaceutical Headquarters—Country
11. Crestor (rosuvastatin)	AstraZeneca LP/ Shionogi & Company	Hypercholes- terolemia	United Kingdom/ Sweden/Japan
12. Coreg (carvedilol)	Glaxo SmithKline	Hypertension	United Kingdom
13. Avandia (rosiglitazone)	Glaxo SmithKline	Diabetes mellitus	United Kingdom
14. Flovent (fluticasone)	Glaxo SmithKline	Asthma	United Kingdom
15. Advair (fluticasone-salmeterol)	Glaxo SmithKline	Asthma	United Kingdom
16. Valtrex (valacyclovir)	Glaxo SmithKline	Herpes	United Kingdom
17. Paxil (paroxetine)	Glaxo SmithKline	Depression	United Kingdom
18. Lovenox (enoxaparin)	Aventis	Anticoagu- lation	France
19. Allegra (fexofenadine)	Aventis	Allergies	France
20. Amaryl (glimepiride)	Aventis	Diabetes mellitus	France

Please note that some of these drugs may have been developed in other countries—including the United States.

antihistamine developed and manufactured in Belgium but sold in the United States by Pfizer). I was particularly interested in this drug because none of the R&D costs associated with developing and testing the drug could be linked to Pfizer's bottom line. Though you might assume this drug was discovered by Pfizer (through their multibillion-dollar development program), it was in fact developed and manufactured in Belgium.

Anraud Denis, investor relations manager at UCB, told me: "The public cost per tablet is EUR 1.95 for Zyrtec in the US; in Europe the average price is EUR 0.56." So why are we paying almost four times more for Zyrtec here than they are in Europe?

As I mentioned near the beginning of this chapter, another area of great concern to me—where there is too cozy a connection between medicine and the drug industry—are those instances where powerful physicians control entire medical-school departments and also are paid advisors for pharmaceutical companies. Perhaps the best book to date on this alarming state of affairs is Thomas J. Moore's *Deadly Medicine*. This book details the interactions between leading physicians, the pharmaceutical industry, and the FDA. Moore claims that these interactions may have resulted in the deaths of thousands of patients who took a drug that perhaps should have never been approved for their type of heart disease.[28] (These types of risks are described more fully in Chapter 4, "Should I Get a Second Opinion?" and Chapter 5, "Should I Take Part in a Scientific Study?")

The financial ties between the pharmaceutical industry and physicians working and teaching at the university remain far too close. (The industry influence on physicians conducting patient studies has been outlined in Chapter 5.) Essentially, the physician is rewarded by the industry with financial payments for every patient enrolled in a study. One episode that particularly disturbed me occurred in 1999, when I was invited along with a number of other cardiologists to hear a talk by a leading heart-failure expert at a hotel in New York City. We were offered $500 each to attend the lecture. While there, we heard what I felt was a very biased presentation in favor of a new drug for heart failure called Coreg.

Moreover, in his presentation, the speaker let it slip that he was on the FDA advisory committee that advocated approval for the drug. So here we have a situation where many of the physicians making decisions for the FDA about whether or not to approve a drug for use in the United States are receiving funds from the pharmaceutical company whose medication they are reviewing. Imagine if a general of the United States Air Force was receiving hundreds of thousands of dollars from Boeing as a consultant and at the same time was responsible for picking the next generation of Air Force fighters. How can doctors be allowed to do what no one else should be allowed to do—make biased decisions (worth billions of dollars and perhaps thousands of people's lives) in favor of companies they work for?

Incidentally, this same speaker was recently quoted in *USA Today*, stating that the pharmaceutical companies do not unduly influence most physicians conducting studies.[29]

Essentially, Coreg is a type of beta-blocker, although it has one other unproven property—known as an alpha-blocker. Proponents of Coreg claim that it is the addition of the alpha-blocker property that makes the drug special. Yet studies in the 1980s like the Veterans Administration Heart Failure Trial (VHEFT), showed alpha-blockers to be ineffective in the treatment of chronic heart failure.[30] In addition, if you remember from earlier in this chapter, in the ALLHAT trial the only part of the study stopped prematurely (incidentally, because heart failure was increased by 50 percent in those patients) involved those patients on an alpha-blocker drug (doxazocin, in that case). So I ask what is so magical or special about Coreg? The price! Now while Coreg is indeed very helpful for many patients with heart failure, similar drugs costing only 2 percent as much per dose have not been studied in randomized trials conducted by Coreg's manufacturer (Glaxo SmithKline).

Studies in the 1980s showed that beta-blockers such as Inderal, metoprolol, and atenolol also prolonged life in patients with heart attacks, yet most of these drugs have never been incorporated in the recent trials on heart failure. (Metoprolol was studied in patients in heart failure and was found not to significantly diminish mortality.) The reason for this is because there are no patents on the older drugs and thus the few companies that still manufacture them do so for pennies per dose. Thus no one has a financial incentive to fund an expensive trial.

The manufacturer of Coreg has taken my colleagues and me to some very expensive restaurants. But generic drug companies do not have the resources to market their competing drugs like the big companies—Pfizers, Mercks, AstraZenecas and, in this case, Glaxo SmithKline. I had resisted these dinners for many years, but as part of my investigation I began taking part in these outings. At most, a few minutes are taken to discuss the drug during dinner. While I've never been persuaded by the drug company arguments, many other doctors are being persuaded to use a more expensive brand-name drug.

I must add that in an unusual twist a study known as the COMET trial, comparing Coreg to the much less expensive beta-blocker metoprolol, was recently completed for the treatment of heart failure. That trial did show that compared to immediate release metoprolol (a drug previously shown not to diminish mortality in heart failure patients), Coreg did substantially reduce the incidence of mortality.[31] Thus I must say that Coreg is a good drug for patients with heart failure, but whether it is better than other similar drugs, save for metoprolol, remains to be answered. Whether it is substantially more expensive than the others is very clear. And that it is certainly no better than a water pill costing pennies a day when used in patients for blood pressure control remains certain. For now the FDA has given approval to two beta-blockers for the use in patients with heart failure. One is Coreg and the other is Toprol. Toprol is significantly less costly than Coreg.

One final note on Coreg. Beta-blockers are also very effective medications for hypertension. Recently, I went to the website Drugstore.com to compare the price of Coreg and atenolol, the latter, as noted, available as a generic drug. Both are approved for the use in high blood pressure and equally effective. A six-month supply of Coreg, taken twice a day, costs $526.52. A comparable supply of atenolol (brand name Tenormin) costs less than $12 (based on a maximum suggested daily dose in a patient weighing over 187 lbs., according to Drugstore.com). And atenolol has real advantages over Coreg: It is a once-a-day medication, and it is less likely to cause wheezing and depression. Yet I continue to encounter patients taking Coreg solely for high blood pressure. Moreover, the drug reps who call on me ask me to prescribe it for hypertension, saying, you guessed it, "Well, their insurance company will pay for it." Needless to say, there are no drug reps from the firms producing generic drugs like atenolol out there taking doctors to dinner at four-star bistros or paying them thousands of dollars to give biased lectures to their friends. There is only one reason that a drug costing ten, twenty, or even fifty times more than another drug of comparable efficacy is prescribed more often than the inexpensive medication. By now, you know the answer as well as I do.

Given everything you have read, I am sure you are wondering how you can keep the cost of your medications to a minimum and continue to receive the best medication available. If you have a prescription plan, for the most part generic drugs are either free to you or require a small copayment. Nongeneric medications often require significant copays of as much as $20 to $30 per prescription. Thus, you should tell your doctor to give you (if it is available) the generic equivalent. If you don't have a prescription plan as part of your health-care insurance, here are several ways of minimizing your cost.

First, ask your physician if there are equivalent medications available that are either less costly or generic. Particularly when it comes to hypertension, *newer* certainly does not mean *better.*

There are no studies showing that some of the most expensive and newest drugs for high blood pressure are any better than a diuretic, a generic beta-blocker, or a generic ACE inhibitor (captopril, lisinopril, or enalapril). Many of these drugs can be purchased for less than $10 a month. Similar medications used in heart failure, arthritis, and asthma cost several times more if they are newer and not available as generic medications.

If you need a medication that is not available as a generic brand, then there are still several ways of cutting your cost. Usually your physician has sample medications in his office that are given to him gratis by the drug reps in the hopes that he'll reach for their drug and then prescribe it. In my practice, if a patient tells me he cannot afford a medication, I attempt to give him a one-month supply of samples. In a year I might give a person in need several months of sample medications.

Get a pill cutter. The idea of pill splitting exclusively to cut costs for the hospital or pharmaceutical plans is quite controversial. The American Pharmaceutical Association and the American Medical Association, as well as other organizations, have taken positions against the idea of mandatory drug splitting. While this is the case for institutions, it should not hamper you from doing so. I would just ask your physician and pharmacist if they think it is safe, and of course, I would limit pill splitting to pills, not capsules.

In 1999, the Veterans' Hospital in Tampa, Florida, began a program of pill splitting. The patients were given pill cutters and instructed on how to use them. According to a VA report, within six months over 40 percent of patients were splitting their pills (in this case, simvastatin), and by the end of the year almost 80 percent. Having patients split this one drug saved the hospital $3.5 million a year.[32]

When the investigators looked into the effect of pill splitting they found that those patients who split their pills actually had lower levels of cholesterol than those who did not.

Dr. Randall Stafford, a researcher at the Stanford Center for Research in Disease Prevention, recently published a paper discussing the huge potential cost savings when pill splitting was used properly. Medications like Viagra (50 percent savings), Lipitor (33 percent savings), and Celexa (46 percent savings) were among the many medications he reviewed and found quite safe and effective if cut correctly by patients.[33]

It is unusual for a 20-mg dose of a medication to cost twice as much as a 10-mg pill. Instead, doubling the dose often only means a 20 percent or so higher cost. Unfortunately, many of the pills are no longer scored (made with an indentation down the middle of the pill) because the pharmaceutical companies don't want you to cut your pills. In fact, companies like Merck have begun making some of their pills in such asymmetric shapes that it might be hard for you to cut the pill in even halves. However, a pill cutter can usually do a very good job and they are sold in most pharmacies.

Here are examples of pills and their prices. Imagine you are taking 10 mg of a blood-pressure medication named Zestril. The cost of this pill is $51.83 for a thirty-day supply of the 10-mg pill, but only $54.83 for a thirty-day supply of the 20-mg pill. By purchasing the 20-mg pill and cutting it in half you have lowered your cost by almost 50 percent. Get your doctor to give you a two-week sample of the 20-mg pill every two months, and your cost is now reduced from about $1.40 per pill (for the 10-mg pill) to 75¢ per pill (for the cut 20-mg pill), to under 40¢ a pill if you include the free samples. Even better, the generic version of this pill (which is probably the most important medication to take for heart failure) will soon be available. I learned this after I noticed that the companies were no longer supplying samples of the drug. When I asked the reps of these two companies (drugs manufactured by both Merck and AstraZeneca) why they were no longer bringing in samples, they all replied, as if in unison, "Oh, the drug is going generic."

As I was finishing up this chapter, a generic version of lisinopril did become available. A ninety-day supply of 20-mg tablets of lisinopril is listed at $51.52 on Drugstore.com. So if you cut your pills in half you can get 10 mg of lisinopril (one of the best medications for high blood pressure, heart failure, and diabetic kidney disease) for less than 30¢ per day.

Claritin, also known as loratidine (made by Schering-Plough), is a medication used by millions of allergy sufferers. It has also gone generic and, better yet, is available over the counter (meaning you don't need a prescription). Again, I knew the patent on the drug was about to run out when I noticed we were no longer getting free samples from the company, the reps stopped talking up Claritin, and finally Schering labs came out with the new-and-improved version, called Clarinex. Or so the company says.

The OTC (over-the-counter) version of the drug will cost much less than its competitors, Allegra (Aventis), Clarinex, and Zyrtec (Pfizer). Essentially, the OTC version will be as effective as all the rest and less sedating than Pfizer's drug, Zyrtec. Interestingly, Zyrtec (a drug manufactured by a pharmaceutical company in Belgium and sold by Pfizer in the United States under a licensing agreement) is an old-style sedating antihistamine. In spite of Zyrtec's shortcomings, and because of Pfizer's great marketing department, revenues for Zyrtec were $1.1 billion last year.[34]

What's ironic here is that the over-the-counter medicine could be more expensive than the brand-name drug if you have a prescription plan. Let's say you have a $10 copay for prescription drugs, then the Clarinex would only cost you $10 out of pocket while the same month's supply of OTC Claritin would cost you almost $30. According to an article released by Reuters on February 5, 2003, some insurers have already caught on to that game. Wellpoint Health Networks, a California-based insurer with 13 million members, has already sent out coupons enabling patients to obtain Wyeth's Alavert (OTC loratadine) at $11 a month for one year. It's also boosting the usual $10 copay its clients must pay for the three other prescription drugs. If sales of these three prescription drugs don't plummet this allergy season, then we truly need to blame the consumers and the physicians for it.

It is beyond the scope of this book and frankly not my goal to discuss why medications in Canada or in fact in every other country in the world are less expensive than they are in the United States. We've all heard of Americans purchasing medications abroad, and for some I guess it is an alternative. For those interested in learning about these issues, I suggest you read from the testimony of Alan Sager, Ph.D., before the U.S.

Subcommittee on Consumer Affairs, entitled "Americans Would Save $8 Billion in 2001 If We Paid Canadian Prices for Brand Name Prescription Drugs."[35]

Where are all the great medications the pharmaceutical companies tell us they devote billions of dollars of research to develop? I've already shown you that a simple diuretic first developed some fifty-plus years ago remains the best medication for treating your blood pressure. The best way to reduce risk of a heart attack is by taking aspirin. The only heart-failure medication that makes your heart beat stronger and doesn't kill you was used by Withering in 1785. Beta-blockers (in the form of Inderal), perhaps the best medication to prolong survival in heart failure, have been around since 1967, and angiotensin-converting enzyme inhibitors (like captopril) were synthesized in 1975 and approved by the FDA in the 1980s.

In the September 1999 issue of *The New England Journal of Medicine*, a trial known as the RALES trial studied the effect of the drug spironolactone (also known as Aldactone) on morbidity and mortality in patients with severe heart disease. Sponsored by Searle (since acquired by Pharmacia, which was itself then gobbled up by Pfizer) and originally scheduled to be completed in four years, the study was stopped after two years because of the extraordinary results: spironolactone decreased mortality by 30 percent compared to the placebo.[36] A new wonder drug, right? Wrong. The FDA approved this new wonder drug in December 1959. It has been a generic drug for years and thus no pharmaceutical company had a financial incentive to pay for and sponsor a trial, until 1995. The generic version of this drug can be purchased for just over 20¢ a pill. Yet in spite of this earth-shattering trial, most of us have never heard of the drug, and none of us has watched television commercials or passed billboards hailing it as perhaps the most cost-effective drug (aside from the thiazide diuretic) on the market. That's because it's a generic drug and costs only 20¢ per day.

But if the industry has its way you'll soon see drugs (they are in clinical trials right now) that work just as well as aldactone and perhaps have fewer side effects (about 10 percent of men on aldactone develop slightly enlarged breast size) advertised on TV and in your doctor's office. These "new and better" drugs will probably cost five to ten times more.

All the other drugs tested for heart failure or its associated arrhythmias were either copycat drugs (similar drug made by another manufacturer) or possibly responsible for thousands of premature deaths. Perhaps if the business spent more of its profits on research and not on direct-to-consumer advertisements (over $2.679 billion spent on those "tell your doctor" ads in 2001 alone),[37, 38] they could discover new cures for the countless ailments and diseases that still plague us.

CHAPTER 7

Medicine in Crisis

During the course of writing this book, I have attempted to provide you with the best possible education about the frequently wretched state of modern medicine and, in so doing, to provide the potential medical patient with questions he can ask himself and others in his search of the best care, the best physicians, and the best hospitals this country has to offer. This has frequently involved portraying physicians, hospitals, nurses, the pharmaceutical and insurance industries, medical studies, "best doctors" lists, and whiz-bang technologies in a candid but very harsh light.

I can only imagine that in the process I have shaken the faith of some in a medical system that is in many respects out of control. I regret that this reaction may be an unavoidable consequence of the truth as I see it, for deep down, I still love practicing medicine and I consider it one of the highest callings to which any individual can aspire. Now more than ever, I suppose, one could argue that it is even more important in light of the aging of the baby boomer generation. The pressures this aging process will exert in the next several decades on a system already badly out of whack are nearly incalculable.

In the interest of fairness, I think it would be instructive for you to walk in the shoes of a doctor for a while, or at least to imagine it, and to consider the mind-boggling array of challenges that have conspired to make the practice of medicine in America at the beginning of the third millennium such a hugely daunting challenge every single day. What follows is meant in no way to mitigate any of the issues of vital importance I have raised in previous chapters or to excuse any of the examples of unprofessional, unethical, and dangerous behavior I have decried.

Malpractice

It's no secret that huge malpractice settlements are being awarded to patients every day of the week in America. You would have to be Rip van Winkle himself to be unaware of this fact. With often unscrupulous lawyers and law firms fanning the flames in the Yellow Pages, on radio and television, on billboards and sandwich boards, in leaflets, and on park benches for all I know, the sheer litigiousness of our fellow citizens seems to have reached the proportions of some kind of mass mania, with no end in sight. *Sue first, ask questions later,* seems to be the American mantra these days.

These awards, however, are frequently given by jurors sympathetic to patients who have suffered some form of harm as the result of a treatment, a procedure, a surgery, a medical decision, or a drug regimen even if the result was not brought about by actual malpractice. This is understandable behavior, as no one enjoys hearing about another's suffering, but in reality, this otherwise commendable form of human compassion has been used by a predatory class of attorneys to pervert a system of necessary checks and balances, one that is now out of control and threatening to destroy the practice of medicine as we know it.

We all understand, I think, deep down inside, that our finite and all too brief lives can be subject to uncounted forms of illness, injury, and sudden death. Life, someone once wrote, can be short, brutish, and nasty. Think of the much-loved husband and father who happily throws on his coat and goes out to shovel snow in his driveway and falls dead ten minutes later of a massive heart attack. Or the thirty-year-old woman who dies in childbirth of an extremely rare ruptured aneurysm in her renal artery. Disaster does happen, as much as I hate to admit it, and accepting it is a part of life.

But then why, *why* are doctors and, consequently, our entire health-care system penalized to the brink of financial extinction whenever an unfortunate and very often unavoidable, unpreventable event occurs? The daily threat of such a mind-boggling judgment fills even the very best physicians with terror and, even worse, makes it even more difficult for them to practice the best medicine on their patients. In addition, it gives many physicians an incentive to perform expensive and unwarranted tests on their patients, the justification being that if they do not rule out a cancer or some form of heart disease that they will be blamed for it later and sued for not finding it in the first place.

What is truly ironic about this state of affairs is that many doctors no longer practice medicine the way we were taught to. Or the way we would need to in order to pass our board examination. For example, a thirty-year-old female comes to her doctor's office complaining that she gets a sharp chest pain every time she feels anxious. Should the physician perform a stress test? The correct answer on the exam is no, since the likelihood of this woman's having coronary artery disease is almost nil. Yet, in that one-in-a-million nightmare scenario, what if this woman died of a heart attack shortly after her doctor's visit, during which he or she did not perform the stress test? The lawyers would have a field day. Good-bye home, car, savings account, the whole nine yards. So the physician, acting out of fear and not in response to his or her years of training, thus rationalizes the necessity of performing an unnecessary exam, one costing the woman's insurance company unnecessary expense and in some way contributing to the ever-higher costs of insurance coverage in this country.

The same thing is happening every hour of every day in emergency rooms across this country, where patients are admitted who would never have been admitted before were it not for the fear of a malpractice lawsuit. Healthy young people who come to the local ER with chest pain but who have a normal exam and labs are being admitted to a monitored bed to make sure they're not that one-in-a-million case (and thus the basis for a multimillion dollar lawsuit). Twenty years ago, even ten years ago, patients like this were given reassurance that they were OK and told to go see their doctor if any questions or problems persisted. Now hospitals are frequently filled to capacity with many patients who don't really belong there.

And here is where the line between the fear of legal retribution and the sort of cynicism and greed that I have described begins to blur, for, to make matters even worse, the hospital management tacitly condones these behaviors. Like any good hotelier, the hospital manager's goal is to run his facility with as few vacant rooms as possible, correct? I've been told that in one hospital in New York City the chief of medicine told his doctors to admit more patients since the wards were not nearly full. And in another New York City hospital emergency room, doctors have been told by their administrators to admit patients rather than attempt to make a diagnosis in the ER and then (possibly) send the patient home. No wonder some of you have to wait all day to see a doctor in an ER and then, in instances where you are truly sick enough to be admitted, you must wait to be sent to a hospital bed.

The fear of malpractice has resulted in another unwritten rule: *Don't write anything in the patient's chart that might incriminate you or the hospital down the road.* Doctors are told from the very beginning that the patient's chart is really "a legal document." In fact, a day before starting my internship, my fellow interns and I were forced to sit through a lecture by hospital lawyers who warned us not to write things in the chart that could be used later against us individually or against the hospital in a malpractice suit. We were told to talk about any mishaps or mistakes made in the care of a patient—if the patient gets the wrong medicine or never gets the test that was ordered—but never, under any circumstances, to write it down in the chart.

In spite of this admonition, last year I noted on the chart that a patient of mine did not get appropriate care the night of his admission. I called the covering hospital doctor and had him correct most of the errors. A week later, the vice chairman of medicine at the hospital called me up to tell me that he had received a call from a nursing supervisor, a.k.a. Big Brother, who had copied my note and sent it to him for review. He told me that it was inappropriate to mention anything about the less than adequate care the patient had received and that I was putting the hospital at risk for a lawsuit. He said he understood that the intern had made some stupid mistakes in caring for the patient but insisted that I should have discussed it with the intern and ignored the whole matter in the chart.

You see what I am saying here? That a patient's chart is no longer an accurate or reliable record of the treatment and care he or she has received at a hospital. A chart is a sanitized document at best and untrue to the extent to which information that belongs on it has been withheld. Use a chart in any other way— to tell the unvarnished truth, for example, about a patient's care—and you're considered a traitor to your hospital. This is the environment your physician very often works in: frightened to death of being sued but just as fearful of the consequences of telling the truth on a patient's chart.

Inevitably, no matter how talented, devoted, careful, and even lucky a doctor is, sooner or later he or she will be named in a malpractice suit. I think the average physician probably has to endure four or five of these in his career. (I've been named in one myself, and it was a thoroughly disheartening experience in every way.) Usually the process begins when some stranger arrives at your office to serve you papers in front of your staff and your patients, as if you were some sort of criminal or back-alley abortionist. Your charts and files are copied and sent to the plaintiff's "malpractice attorney."

It just keeps on getting nastier, for the physician doesn't really have his own attorney. He has an attorney assigned to him by his insurance company. This attorney's primary job is to limit the liability of the insurance company and, only secondarily, to protect the physician's interests or reputation. If the plaintiff expresses a willingness to settle the case for $100,000, and the insurance company's attorney feels it is in the best interest of his company to do so, he will strongly urge the doctor to settle and even to admit guilt, even though both the attorney and the doctor realize that no malpractice has been committed.

In other words, the insurance company shells out the $100,000, drastically curtails the amount of time its lawyer spends on the case, and quite possibly limits the company's financial exposure to even greater monetary damages. But what about the doctor? Now his record has been blemished. The settlement and/or admission of guilt becomes part of the state record, and the doctor must report this fact every time he renews his hospital privileges or signs up with a new insurance company (usually with an enclosed description of the case and settlement).

In the largest and most well-publicized cases, huge, immensely powerful, and often intimidating malpractice firms can request millions in payment for their clients' *pain and suffering*. Imagine what it must feel like when you realize that a team of all-star lawyers may soon be squaring off in court with your in-house, salaried, possibly inexperienced, and probably not very loyal insurance attorney. And if your insurance cap is only good for $2 million, then your house might be up for grabs too. So imagine the grip of fear most every doctor, good or bad, has to live with as each attempts to do his job in today's environment. It's downright scary.

I hate to have to say it, by the way, but those two words, *pain* and *suffering*, which define the very things that every conscientious physician sets out to prevent from the very first day of his or her training, are responsible for some truly ridiculous but nonetheless horribly onerous settlements. Even President Bush has recognized the need to limit awards for pain and suffering in his latest package of proposed tort reforms.

But wait a minute. Let's say the doctor wins the lawsuit. "Wins what?" I would counter. After giving a lengthy deposition on the case, the physician is then required by his insurance company to sit in the courtroom for the entire duration of the trial, whether it takes two days, two weeks, or two years. He cannot keep up with the treatment of his patients or the care of his practice. He loses income, as well. But he won the case, right? Wrong. In my view, if you get named in any lawsuit, you lose. And I doubt that a physician has ever sued the malpractice attorney for lost time or earnings in a frivolous suit.

There are, of course, indisputable instances of medical malpractice committed by many physicians in this country (witness the recent, disastrously botched operation on a young girl in North Carolina who was given a heart from a donor with the wrong blood type), but even in such blatant cases the financial compensation awarded can be outrageously enormous. I'm not saying that the physicians who commit such errors in judgment should not be punished or that patients and their families are not deserving of *fair* treatment in the courts. On the contrary, the doctor responsible for the malpractice should be disciplined, fined, suspended, and/or stripped of his or her license to practice medicine. If a hospital is involved, similar injunctions should be applicable.

But the focus should be on preventing future occurrences rather than on the outsized, punitive, and emotionally charged financial rewards given to patients and their lawyers. The system we have now is out of whack and entirely unfair, and I can assure you it will have—already has had—ruinous consequences. Huge settlements for a plaintiff result in higher rates for all doctors, be they good or bad, and many committed physicians are choosing to leave the profession rather than face the expense of ever-rising malpractice insurance or the daily terrors I have described above.

Doctor's Salaries

It might come as a considerable shock to you to learn that not every doctor in this country is a millionaire. That may be the common perception, but the truth is far from it. In fact, if you would just put aside any assumptions you may have acquired over the years, you will quickly see that it is getting harder and harder for physicians to live a comfortable life, to buy a nice house or car, and save for a happy retirement. At the beginning of 2003, physicians in two states either threatened to or actually did go out on strike to make this point. The physician's cost of doing business is increasing exponentially every year, in large part because malpractice premiums have skyrocketed, sometimes to more than $100,000 per year. But unlike most other professions, doctors cannot for the most part increase their prices to make up for these steadily increasing overhead costs.

For the past twenty years or so most of the financial compensation received by physicians has come directly from the insurance companies, with very little out-of-pocket expense for the patient. Doctors who accept this type of insurance—and most of them do—are *told precisely what they can charge* by the insurance company for a given procedure, exam, or office visit, whether the insurer be Medicare, Oxford Health, or some other company. Imagine what would happen if in 1980 General Motors was told by some governing body that it could charge only $20,000 for a Cadillac. I guess they might still be able to make a good car and a decent profit. Yet, imagine that in the year 2003 they were mandated to charge only $17,000 for their new model. The costs of materials and labor have no doubt risen year by year, and, to make matters worse, let's say that because the attorneys of our country had declared open season on the company that GM has had to pay out billions of dollars in order to settle lawsuits, many of which were truly unfounded. I suspect that General Motors would declare bankruptcy, forgo reorganization, and close shop for good. This is the atmosphere in which many physicians are doing business: increasing overhead and mandated declining compensation for their services. Why would any sane business-person enter into such a line of work?

But there is more. Imagine what it is like to start the first day of your career with a couple of hundred thousand dollars of debt. Four years of college and another four years of medical school can leave a recent graduate with up to $250,000 in loans.

And unlike someone with a new law degree or MBA, doctors only earn about $40,000 a year during the time they work in a residency program. If you entertain the ambition of becoming a gastroenterologist or cardiologist, you'll be working like a dog at that salary for another six or seven years.

As I mentioned before, reimbursements for procedures and exams have significantly diminished in the past ten years, sometimes by as much as 50 percent. This is in the face of an increased cost of housing and living and a substantial increase in malpractice insurance. So how do doctors survive?

Well, some physicians survive by performing more tests and accepting "bribes" in the form of phantom rents, drug-company dinners, and other under-the-table payments. Add the other mammoth incentive—"If I miss something, they'll sue me"—and you have the simplest explanation of why there are too many procedures done in our country and why the cost of medicine and your insurance premiums are out of control.

Some physicians decide against clinical practice and work for a university hospital as a faculty doctor. Yet, the hospitals are caught in the same tightening vice as the physicians are: increasing costs and decreasing payments. Salaries at a university hospital for full-time physicians have not increased for years, and many doctors are therefore pressed to earn additional money elsewhere. Most of these full-time physicians remain honest and hardworking, but some, driven by their diminutive salaried positions, become spokespersons for the pharmaceutical companies. And these people are the very physicians often responsible for teaching new doctors. We've read about the physician who "doubled" his salary "lecturing" for pharmaceutical companies. That same doctor rarely prescribes less-expensive generic drugs that offer the same results as the expensive drugs manufactured by the company he lectures for.

I've said this before, but it is worth repeating. By means of lecture fees, grants, and payments to physicians who enroll patients in studies, the huge pharmaceutical companies have insinuated themselves into every nook and cranny of the medical community. In this case, they manipulate hardworking and perhaps financially hard-pressed physicians into promoting their drugs to physicians in the community and/or to residents in training. I would be willing to bet that nearly 90 percent of young academic physicians also work for pharmaceutical companies.

I think this unfair system of rewards has helped create some of the greed we now see in medicine, and I have no doubt that at least some of the physicians who are involved in improper moneymaking schemes that defraud you and our health-care system would not be doing so if they had been properly compensated for their work.

The Exams

Do you know how many national board exams—many now costing about $1,000 each—a qualified physician needs to pass during his or her career? You might be surprised. In medical school students must pass the national boards, part one and part two, in order to graduate. Then, during their internship, they must pass the third part of the boards. During their residency, they must take and pass an internal medicine exam for residents-in-training. On completion of their training, they must pass the Internal Medicine Board exam to get board certification—and then pass it again every ten years. If you go into a specialty, like cardiology, pulmonology, etc., you must pass that exam in order to become board certified and then retake a home exam and sit for the board exam every ten years if you wish to continue to be board certified. If you want to get certified in angiogram, echo, nuclear cardiology, or arrhythmia, you also must take that exam every ten years. It adds up. The elderly physicians who might have fallen out of touch with modern methods are exempt from taking these exams.

The HMO

I think I participate in about twenty different health maintenance organizations now. Every year or two, depending on the HMO, I am asked to fill out a new application in order to renew my participation. They all ask essentially the same questions: where I went to school and/or trained, have I been convicted of a crime or involved in a lawsuit, etc. Why, I have to wonder, is such a tedious and time-consuming process necessary?

But that's not all the paperwork you need to get through once you are a member of an HMO. Not if you want to get paid for your services. There are calls to make and forms to fill out and then get approved before you can perform just about any test in your office or even send a patient for a CAT scan or MRI. And when members of our staff call the HMO 800 number they often are put on hold for as long as you are when you call your local cable company. If they make twenty or more calls like that in a day, you have a staff pretty close to mutiny. Things got so bad in my office that my exhausted and frustrated staff pleaded with me to turn over our paperwork to a private billing company. Rather than see our staff continue to suffer the consequences of modern medical red tape, not to mention a bout of major depression (and I'm serious about this), my colleagues and I tossed out a $20,000 billing system and hired an outside company (which naturally takes about 6 percent of our collections for their fee).

In addition to these bureaucratic hassles, many doctors and patients have been punished by the sometimes thoughtless and frankly stupid policies of an HMO. For example, in January 2001, the American College of Physicians released a statement concerning an HMO in Muskegon, Michigan. The people that run this HMO decided to force members to stop using doctors of internal medicine as primary-care physicians, even if the doctor was a member of the HMO. The HMO demanded they use a family practitioner or general practitioner solely as their primary doctor. In doing this they attempted to destroy the practices of many internists, who really function as general practitioners for adults, and to sever long-standing doctor/patient relationships as well, all based on the probably erroneous assumption that they could improve their profit margins.[1] Less than one week later, after hearing numerous concerns from plan members, physician partners, and medical societies, the HMO reversed its policy.

If an HMO ever attempts to implement these types of policy changes in connection with your coverage or benefits, I would threaten to cancel your policy with them and report the HMO to your state attorney general. If you do cancel your policy, just ask your doctor to recommend a policy for you, or at least to give you a list of the HMOs of which he is a member.

To help keep pharmacy costs as manageable as possible, most HMOs have created incentives for us to use generic drugs. Frankly, I think it is a good idea to keep costs down. A generic drug is essentially an exact duplicate of the more expensive brand-name medication, so for me the switch is easy. However, when insurance companies begin to discount (to their insured members) what they consider to be the preferred drug (a drug that is cheaper), I begin to question the efficacy of that drug.

In my plan, a generic brand of a medication only costs me $7, while a preferred brand costs $20 and a nonpreferred brand $40. Unlike generic drugs, however, these preferred drugs, while usually in the same drug class, are not all alike. Each drug is metabolized differently. Moreover, each drug interacts with other medications differently and, as I showed you with the cholesterol-lowering drug Zocor and blood-thinning Coumadin, sometimes dangerously. One brand of a blood-pressure medication might cause swelling of the ankles far more often than another, or another might elevate or lower the levels of other drugs you are taking already. And there are those people who for whatever reason cannot tolerate the preferred brand of medication. Being forced to pay $40 a month for each nonpreferred brand is like not having insurance at all. So while I applaud the idea of encouraging the use of generic drugs, I don't think we should allow insurers to dictate which brand-name drugs we use. That's just too dangerous a practice.

In the defense of the HMO system, I should point out that they do manage to do a reasonable job at holding down the cost of health care, while at the same time asserting an admirable degree of quality control, unlike Medicare, which is just plain out of control in both of these areas. HMOs insist, for example, that doctors be certified to do special consultations or to perform special tests, such as echocardiograms or colonoscopies, if they wish to get paid for them.

An HMO official will often audit a chart, request records, and sometimes even call to ask a physician why a test needs to be done. When someone on the phone seems at first blush to be second-guessing a decision you have made or one you want to carry out in the middle of busy office hours or while you are seeing patients in the hospital, it can be a royal pain. But I also understand why they have to do it. And the good news, of course, is that they employ people smart enough and educated enough to make such inquiries in the first place. Without someone to watch over a doctor's decisions, way too many tests would be done, for all the reasons I have articulated elsewhere in this book.

Medicare, however, is far more lenient in this regard, and thus it allows many unqualified doctors—who are actually criminals, in my view—to perform all sorts of tests they are not qualified or trained to perform or interpret. Therefore, under the Medicare rules, the quality of patient care suffers at the very same time that the costs of maintaining the program are skyrocketing. A lose/lose situation if ever there was one.

In response to President Bush's State of the Union Address,

where he suggested the privatization of Medicare, Robert M. Hayes, president of the nonprofit Medicare Rights Center, said, "The problem is not Medicare's structure, which works better than any private marketplace structure to ensure universal coverage and access to health care people need. The problem is Medicare needs a prescription drug benefit."[2] He couldn't be more wrong. Medicare needs to be overhauled or replaced by another means of delivering cost-effective care for those who use it.

The Plight of the Private Doctor

In 1990, I decided I had had enough of taking orders from some very unpleasant and manipulative faculty physicians at Montefiore Medical Center, and so at the request of the hospital's president, Spencer Foreman, I decided, with a colleague, to open a private practice, one that allowed us to make our own decisions, even while we still maintained an affiliation with Montefiore. The idea of a hospital encouraging a couple of recent graduates to open their own office was so novel that we were featured on the front page of *Crain's Business News* (actually there was a photo of the president of the hospital on the cover, but our names were at least mentioned). The hospital's idea was to allow us to grow a quality practice in a suburban area only a few miles from Montefiore and therefore refer new patients for cardiac catheterization, pacemakers, and surgery, the big-money earners for any hospital. In return, the hospital granted us a loan at reasonable rates and gave us some free advice. Strangely enough, I never spoke with or met Spencer Foreman during this process.

Things went well for us, and we slowly built up our practice. We took a very small salary for the first two years, and my partner, who was married, worked in the local ER twice a week in order to support his family. At first, many of the hospital nurses and staff were helpful and encouraged patients to come see us. As the volume of our practice grew, however, reimbursements from the insurance companies began to shrink, and things changed. The hospital's cardiology department now more than ever needed more money to balance their budget. So, suddenly, nurses who worked for the cardiology department at the hospital were told not to send any patients to our practice. We had known some of the nurses since the days of our residency, but they all complied with the orders they had been given and stopped referring patients to us. To their credit, some of them came to me and told me that their superiors had told them to stop referring patients to physicians not employed by the hospital. They were told that the full-time employed physicians (the doctors who get paid directly by the hospital) needed the money. So from that day forward, we never received a patient from any of the cardiology nurses. This is the environment that many private physicians who are affiliated with large medical centers have to contend with. In return, these same private physicians, often called voluntary physicians, are still required to teach the students and residents affiliated with the hospital for up to two months of the year and to do it for free.

The Patients

The environment in the physician's office has also changed. Perhaps this is because of the bad press doctors have gotten over the years or the 1-800-SUE YOUR DOCTOR advertisements festooned all over the highways and media, or perhaps it is because we don't do such a great job caring for patients anymore. I don't know. But imagine for a moment, no matter what your profession—plumber, accountant, banker, teacher, whatever—what it would be like if you were the target of advertisements strewn all over the highway by a group of lawyers (1-800-SUE YOUR PLUMBER, or ACCOUNTANT, or BANKER, or TEACHER)? How would that affect your public image? And your state of mind? I can tell you that every physician is noticing a loss of respect from his or her patients.

I'm talking about simple things like patients not showing up for a scheduled appointment. In my practice, I'd say that about 10 percent to 20 percent of patients not only don't show up but also lack the courtesy to call and explain why they cannot make their appointment. This form of disrespect plays havoc with our schedules, needless to say, but that is the least of it. Nuclear stress tests, for example, require us to order expensive radioactive doses in advance. We call patients the day before to remind them of the test, yet even with this reminder, very often they don't show up. We therefore end up having to absorb the cost of this wasted dosage, as patients always refuse to pay.

Two years ago I received what had to be the best reply to the question I always ask my patients when I see them after they have failed to show up or call for their last appointment. "Why," I asked a patient, "did you not show up for your last appointment?"

She replied, angrily, I might add, "It was not my fault. I forgot!"

Top-notch medical care should by no means be a commodity available only for the wealthy, but it should not be taken for granted either. It simply is not fair that doctors have no ability to bill a patient who misses an appointment (sometimes appointment after appointment) and who lacks the courtesy to let us know in advance. At first, when confronted with a no-show patient, many physicians just sat idly in the office for that blank half hour and waited for the next patient to show up. Now most of us have taken the approach of the airlines or hotels: overbook by 10 percent. So on the rare day when all the patients show up, they will have to wait for an hour or more to see the doctor.

I'm not saying you should sit in a waiting room for hours. In fact, in that instance, I would certainly leave. I might even consider finding another doctor. But I hope you can appreciate why a doctor can't see you within thirty minutes of your appointment time on occasion.

It is inappropriate for patients to call their doctor late at night or on a weekend because they have run out of their medication or to ask a simple, nonemergency question or to call to discuss the care of their relative. Doctors are there 24/7 for emergencies but not for casual talk, nonurgent questions, or calling in refills that should have been taken care of during office hours.

Abusive demands from patients can be taxing too. A urologist recently told me a story about a demented, bedridden, dying patient he was called to see at the nursing home where he consults. The doctor caring for the patient had called the urologist to administer a drug called Lupron (at $1,000 per shot) for the patient's prostate cancer. The urologist correctly felt that it was unethical to continue such injections for this patient and wrote as much in his consult. A day later he received a call from the family of the patient, warning him that if their dad did not get his shot they would report him to the Office of Professional Misconduct. The risk and the hassle associated with such a spurious report were such that the doctor went ahead, against his principles and better judgment, and gave the patient his shot.

Disability: Forms and Abuse

Could you guess how much a physician receives for filling out an eight-page disability form? In New York State, physicians receive $10. Imagine if the disability lawyers were required to accept $10 for filling out their part of this densely worded document.

To make matters worse, some of the patients my colleagues and I see want more disability time than they deserve. A patient might have a mild heart attack and require a couple of weeks to recuperate before he goes back to his desk job. Yet many patients, in my experience, have tried to coax me into giving them months off instead of the perhaps one or two weeks they deserve. Some patients, I believe, have left our practice to look for another physician who will continue to designate them as disabled. In one specific case, we were able to diagnose and rush into surgery a man with a deadly heart ailment. A few weeks later, the fellow came to the office to thank me for saving his life. The next week, however, he was back to complain, most vociferously, that I would not designate him as disabled for the rest of his life. He subsequently went as far as hiring a disability attorney to see if he could arrange something.

It is not the case that good doctors don't believe in designating patients as disabled when they are disabled. Some doctors, however, in response to a kind of implied blackmail, will designate a patient as disabled rather than send him to another doctor. My dad worked two jobs and seven days a week to keep his family warm and fed, so this type of spurious claim really bothers me.

We All Have to Play the Game. Or Do We?

Most honest doctors know what is going on all around them: who is doing illegal and unethical things, performing tests and procedures for which they are not qualified, touting for the big pharmaceutical companies, etc. Yet, no one talks. Well, until now, anyway.

Sometimes, if I know a patient well enough and I see he is being treated by an unscrupulous doctor, I tell him so. I tell him when I know that tests ordered by his other physician are either inappropriate or cannot be accurately interpreted by the physician in question. I will even tell him to find another doctor pronto and never return to his old one.

But I know very few other doctors who do so, and I wonder what that says about my profession. I am well aware that it is far easier in life to take the path of least resistance, to turn a blind eye, just like the self-serving Sergeant Schultz in the sixties TV show *Hogan's Heroes*. Perhaps there are many physicians who not only know of an unscrupulous doctor or unscrupulous practices but have also actually gotten into bed with them. The bad apple just might be sending the other MD lots of work.

Let me give you an example from my own practice. For a few years I'd been treating a gentleman with a rapid heartbeat in my office. His wife would usually come with him, and we all got to know one another. They're simple folks, blue-collar types dressed in jeans and sweatshirts (with a Yankees logo on them) and very friendly to me and my staff.

One day they told me they were also seeing a general practitioner (GP) and that the GP had found a leak in the wife's heart valve. The doctor also said that she had bladder polyps and should see a specialist for that and that both of them should undergo a colonoscopy. He also told my patient to go see a urologist because he probably needed testosterone injections. Every physician I know would have nodded his head and just focused on the patient's primary reason for visiting him. But my heart wouldn't let me do that. I felt great sympathy for these rather naïve but fine folks, and I did not want to see them frightened or taken advantage of.

I was also acquainted with the GP in question and knew him to be a shrewd businessman but not someone I could recommend as a good doctor. For starters, I quickly established that the man's wife had been given an echocardiogram by a portable radiology service that rented space from that same doctor (the doctor who ran that service subsequently had his medical license suspended by the New York State health commissioner). Furthermore, she had been given the test for no reason. She did not have a murmur.

Thus, I closed the exam-room door and asked them if they trusted me. When they said they did, I told them never to see their GP again. I sent them to other doctors who found nothing wrong with them; there was no need for constant injections of testosterone or the colonoscopies. Afterward, they asked that unscrupulous doctor to send their patient records to me. I don't think our office ever did get those records, but my partner did get a call.

The doctor reminded him that he was a GP and would love to send patients to us, but that Dr. Levine seemed to be taking over the care of his patient. I don't think we've seen a patient from that doctor since. But I wouldn't have it any other way.

Here's another one of my favorite true stories. When I first opened my private practice, I met, usually over lunch, many of the physicians who practiced at one or another of the small hospitals we admit to. After a month of this, they invited me to their weekly card game.

The game was a high-stakes game of poker, seven-card stud, with many opportunities to bet on a hand. They played with several wild cards, making even an otherwise great hand like a full house easy to beat. In any event, I lost a few hundred dollars that night, but as I left I was told I would have a consult the next day to make up for my loss. The next morning I was called to clear an eighty-five-year-old nursing-home patient for his operation, a penile implant. I never played cards with those physicians again and for the most part never spoke with them again either.

If you were a physician, what would you do in the following situation? I saw a gentleman recently with a chronic arrhythmia, called atrial fibrillation, that had probably caused a stroke on the left side of his body two years ago. He had seen a stomach doctor who was so concerned about the quality of the patient's care that he asked the patient to speak to me later that afternoon.

The patient had been seeing a GP for the past two years. The patient and his wife told me that his doctor's technician, who comes to his office once a week, had performed a sonogram of his neck, heart, and abdomen a few weeks before. I asked why all these tests had been done, and she told me that the doctor was a specialist in this area. In fact, this physician had no experience or training in these complex studies.

When I asked them how often he was checking the gentleman's blood-thinner levels (Coumadin level), they told me about three times per year. Coumadin needs to be checked at least as often as once a month. Finally, I asked if the doctor had discussed what foods the man should avoid; foods with lots of vitamin K, like green vegetables, counteract the effects of Coumadin. They told me that he had never discussed a special diet, and when I asked the patient if he ate broccoli, a vegetable with lots of vitamin K, he told me that he ate it just about every night.

So what would you do if you were seeing this patient for the first time? I sat the patient and his wife down and told them the truth. I told them that he had had all those sonogram tests for only one reason: to fill the pockets of the doctor who did them. Then I repeated his sonogram for free, since I know that the insurance company, having paid his GP for the same study, would not pay me, and I told them not to worry about it.

I checked his Coumadin level and found it dangerously low. I changed his Coumadin as well as his other medications and told him never to return to that doctor again. I gave him a list of other internists to see, but I could not refuse his tearful wife's plea that I see him next week. Finally, I tried to call his insurance company's fraud line, but they were not interested.

Please make sure you, your friends, and your family do not get suckered by a similarly corrupt and greedy physician.

Over the past few years I had received many consults from that doctor. But once he heard that his patient had left him, and had done so after seeing me, he would not send any more consults to our practice. I called my partners that night and told them that I just could not let the elderly man and his wife go back to that doctor.

Now imagine taking the other approach, like so many businesspeople do, and selling your soul for the right price. Doctors are after all in "business to practice medicine." Ignoring the immoral behaviors of doctors like the ones I describe, taking them to dinner, and giving them a pat on the back when you see them could help create a relationship worth perhaps $100,000 a year to you. What would you do if your livelihood depended on it?

Free Dinners and Trips

As I have written elsewhere in this book, the pharmaceutical companies are eager to take physicians to a lavish dinner or to send them on a junket masquerading as a seminar. They target physicians with large practices, specialists who prescribe expensive drugs, physicians with influence over those in training, or experts in the field. When I first began my practice I went on many dinners and gave unbiased talks about specific diseases or drugs. I'm an outgoing person and a good public speaker, but many of the companies did not ask me back since I gave the speech I wanted to give and not the one-sided version the companies had hoped for.

Frankly, as far as these dinners were concerned, I quickly realized that they were not for me. I did not wish to feel that I owed someone or some corporation something in return. Not going to these free dinners, however, was without question bad for business. Physicians who consistently attend these dinners and seminars develop relationships with other doctors as well as with the drug companies. These events prove a fertile place in which to market and grow your practice. After several years of turning down these dinners, my colleagues and I have begun to go out again with the reps and other doctors, and we have increased our practice size because of it. I feel hypocritical going to these dinners, but I don't go often and I never change my prescribing pattern because of them.

The Good Doctors

In spite of all the temptations and the hardships, as a group, physicians should be among the most honored people of our society. There are so many caring and special people who practice medicine even today, people whom I've met over the past twenty years, both professors and clinicians. Doctors like Leticia Gonzales and her associates, who could probably earn twice as much income if they performed all sorts of sonography studies or rented their office in a phantom rent scheme. Or the doctors in the Beth Abraham Geriatrics Group, who work for a relatively small salary yet never seem to tire of or to question their work with the elderly.

It's worth pointing out here that I do not know of another profession whose practitioners routinely expect to work for no compensation, but in the medical field this is an unavoidable fact of life—one that most every doctor I know accepts with grace and out of a genuine desire to help his fellow man. When patients are admitted to the hospital without insurance, someone has to take care of them, even though physicians risk a malpractice suit every time they see a nonpaying patient. Patients who have no insurance or who are covered only by Medicaid are sometimes uneducated, less likely to follow the requirements of their medications and diet. Thus, they are very difficult to care for, and often arrive in the hospital in pretty dreadful shape with conditions that could have easily been avoided. Most hospitals have call schedules in each different department (medicine, surgery, etc.) for just this reason. Doctors call it their *service time*. Sometimes physicians will even take service calls for a month at a time and turn it into a doubly positive use of their time by teaching and reviewing these service cases with the medical students and residents in training. If it were not for such doctors, these individuals would have no health care of any kind. But I am proud to say that most of us take care of these patients for free when we are on service.

But based on the way our health-care system works today, those physicians with the greatest integrity are struggling to pay their bills or perhaps cannot afford a nice home for their family. Even worse, perhaps, is the constant pressure to do the wrong thing because they see the dishonest physicians drive up to the hospital in a 500-class Mercedes. I'm hoping that this book embarrasses those physicians who are involved in the scandals I've brought up and somehow rewards those many good doctors with whom I've enjoyed working and who I know practice honorable medicine.

Conclusion

know that what I have written will shock some readers. You may have learned more than you wanted to about a once-venerable institution. Medicine in this country—how it is practiced and paid for—might be on the critical list. But my intention has never been to frighten or alarm but rather to inform and educate. It is always the best-informed, best-educated consumer, no matter what the product or service may be, who will receive the best products and services. And who can always insist on receiving them. It can be no different when it comes to the vast medical marketplace, and I am convinced that if you stick with my suggestions, you'll be much better able to avoid the dangers. Moreover, you'll be able to take genuine comfort in also being able to help your loved ones, especially those who are either too sick or too young or too old to help themselves, just as I have been able to help members of my own family.

So, what about some remedies? How can we fix our pharmaceutical system and how can you get the best medicines at the least cost? For one thing, Congress needs to throw a lasso around the pharmaceutical companies and restrict their ability to charge whatever they like for the drugs they sell to Americans, perhaps in much the same way the European nations have. If the companies argue that price-fixing is anti-American and just as unfair as fixing the prices that doctors can charge their patients, then perhaps serious thought should be given to instituting some sort of universal drug coverage for every American.

But there are other ways that we can help the pharmaceutical companies reduce their costs. I have shown you that these companies spend billions upon billions of dollars marketing their products. So why not restrict all direct-to-consumer marketing? Ban all the television and radio commercials as well as the newspaper and magazine advertisements. Perhaps the Pfizers and Mercks and Abbott Labs might even be willing to formulate voluntary restrictions on such spending.

I would recommend that we abolish the cadres of sales representatives employed by the pharmaceutical companies to "sell" their products. Physicians would no longer have to put up with the pressure tactics, manipulations, and crude, often unethical inducements, and the companies themselves could reduce their overheads by billions of dollars annually. Gone would be the salaries for these people, the free cups and pens, the expensive dinners, honorariums, and trips to resorts masquerading as seminars. If a doctor wanted to obtain samples of a drug or literature about its efficacy, a toll-free number or an Internet website would provide all the necessary information. And perhaps thereafter doctors would prescribe medicines based solely on their merits and efficacy for the individual patient and not because they were the drugs marketed by his or her favorite rep.

I would work to pass legislation that prohibits patients from suing a company for the untoward effects of a drug once the FDA has approved it. All drugs have the potential to cause unanticipated ill effects, but if a panel of experts finds that the studies on a particular drug have been conducted in an honest and professional manner, lawsuits against the manufacturer should be rejected.

I would mandate that the pharmaceutical industry never be allowed to hire any physician currently involved in the FDA's process of approving drugs. In addition, any physician participating in such a process at the FDA should not be allowed to work for a pharmaceutical company for a minimum of three years after his resignation from the panel. To me, this is just common sense.

I would call upon the major medical societies to undergo a process of ethical housecleaning. All too often these institutions allow the pharmaceutical companies and medical device manufacturers to sponsor lectures in their buildings and to fill their publications with advertisements.

Finally, I think the time has come for the government to enact some sort of universal prescription-drug program, which might actually increase the use of prescription drugs and probably be a windfall for the pharmaceutical companies, as much as I hate to admit it.

In return for these huge benefits of both cost reduction and increased sales, some think that a sweeping system of price controls would become obligatory. First, we should require foreign firms that sell or license drugs in the United States not to charge a higher price here for a given drug than they do in their own country or within the European Union. Drugs like Zyrtec and Aricept, while marketed by American companies (in this case, Pfizer) were developed by foreign companies and are sold overseas at a fraction of the cost to consumers in the States. Second, citizens enrolled in the universal prescription program should be given access only to those drugs a special FDA or government panel has approved. In other words, if a generic, and by definition less-expensive, drug is available, then only the generic drug will be available for free to the patient. If you want a brand-name drug still covered by patent protection because you mistakenly believe that it's better, then you'll have to pay for it out of pocket.

How much money could we save as a nation if we lowered our spending on brand-name prescription drugs to the same per-capita amount spent by our Canadian neighbors? Well, according to a presentation given by Dr. Alan Sager on September 5, 2001, to the Subcommittee on Consumer Affairs in Washington, we could have saved $38 billion in 2001.[1] And his estimate does not include the savings that would be achieved by using more generic prescription drugs or by mandating that European drug manufacturers charge us the same as they charge their own citizens for their drugs.

Of course the cadre of lawyers would be against all this, as would the soon-to-be-disenfranchised sales reps, the doctors hungry for perks like expensive meals and vacations, and those unethical physicians who work both sides of the fence. But the rest of us would enjoy a huge benefit. Those with insurance would probably pay less for their premiums, and those without a private-pay prescription plan would be covered under a universal prescription policy.

In the summer of 2003, the cost of prescription drugs and how best to get them to the public—both the elderly with Medicare benefits and the uninsured—was the subject of intense debate in Congress. If you don't know by now, Medicare only pays 80 percent of the medical bills of the elderly, often leaving those without secondary insurance to face huge bills, especially for prescription drugs, which it doesn't pay for at all.

Ironically, those elderly patients who are deemed to be poor also get Medicaid (which pays for the remainder of their medical bills including prescription drugs). The elderly middle class—with even the smallest of savings and without very expensive secondary insurance—is forced to pay out of pocket for the remainder of their care.

It is the hope of many that this Medicaid prescription drug plan can be extended to the elderly. Others, including President Bush and, interestingly, the pharmaceutical industry, argue that private enterprise should be responsible for this total health care package for the elderly. Essentially, this plan suggests that the elderly can opt to join private-pay insurance plans (they would be paid through vouchers otherwise spent by Medicare), which could, through better management, supply full coverage (instead of just medical coverage). The pharmaceutical industry probably prefers this approach because they fear that if the government controls a huge percent of the market (through Medicaid and Medicare drug programs) it might be able to dictate drug prices. As of August 2003, no decision had been made.

In July 2003, however, a momentous decision was made in the House of Representatives, when a vote was passed allowing Americans to import prescription drugs from the EU and Canada. It was a very positive and long overdue step toward realizing a more equitable cost of prescription drugs for Americans. Yet, according to *The New York Times*, fifty-three United States Senators signed a letter opposing this legislation.[2] As you have already read, I think that it is unfair that our citizens often pay twice (if not more) per pill for the same exact medications sold in other countries. I hope that decency will win out over the greed of big business and we will soon have some sort of equality between U.S. prescription-drug costs and the cost of drugs overseas.

Whether or not any of these notions ever becomes a reality, in the here and now it is incumbent upon both health-care providers and patients to keep the cost of prescription drugs as low as possible. Always ask for a generic equivalent to the drug you have been prescribed, or at least for a less-expensive, if equally efficacious, copycat drug. Ask your doctor for as many samples as he or she can afford to spare for you, and finally, go to the trouble of investing in a pill cutter. Remember to ask your doctor and pharmacist if your pills can safely be cut.

I have tried to suggest to you the best ways to locate a good doctor and to maintain a good relationship with him or her. Treat your doctor with some respect, don't abuse the 24/7 rule, and show up on time for your appointments.

If you need to find a specialist, don't go to a relative of your physician, no matter how highly you regard him. Recently a friend of mine told me that he went for a stress test at the office of his internist's brother. Don't do such a thing—ever. Would you send a customer to your brother, wife, or any relative, no matter what their field, if there was a better person for the job in the same town? Of course you wouldn't. And if you are a patient in a multispecialty group and you need an operation or invasive test, go get a second opinion outside of the group. Doctors who practice together almost never disagree with each other; it's just bad politics and creates tension in the partnership.

Don't go to a physician just because he or she seems to be the busiest in town. In my experience, the busiest doctors are very often not the best. Sometimes they are just the best salespeople.

And finally, don't go to clinics unless you absolutely must. Go to a doctor's office. You are a person, not some object that is going to be treated on an assembly line. You want a doctor who is going to be there for you for years to come, not one who changes locations every year or two or who only sees you in the office and not the hospital.

It's unfortunate that hospitals seem to be spending more on advertising these days than on improving patient care. I've told you about the pitfalls of going to the hospital, about the dangers of staying there, and I've given you some advice on how to avoid some deadly mistakes. When I wrote "How to Survive Your Hospital Stay," I truly meant that, but it is more than "surviving," of course, that is in question. At every stage of the process you must strive to limit your exposure to risk—i.e., risk of incompetence, a mistaken diagnosis or poorly inserted intravenous tube, or the laziness and sloth that is all too prevalent in our hospitals today. You must also insist, and if you cannot, your family and friends must insist on your behalf, that you be treated with decency and dignity at all times. You'll need a hard-nosed caring physician to make sure you are not being taken advantage of—enrolled in dangerous studies or discharged before you are ready to go home—and if you are in luck you'll start the process by being admitted to a quality hospital. Though it won't be a matter of luck if you have done your homework first and know where the best teaching hospital is in your area. And before you are admitted there, make sure your own doctor will see you in that facility, and not some stranger or one of the ever more present "hospitalists" many hospitals use these days.

Always remember that you have the final say in every part of your care—even in your preference of a roommate—and never be afraid to call an administrator to complain or, better yet, put your complaint in writing. Any written complaint sent to the president of a hospital is a potential stain on his or her and the hospital's reputation, and frankly it plants the germ of a potential lawsuit in the minds of the hospital administrators, so it will get you some attention and, one hopes, the appropriate action. It is very simple: People who don't complain about the bad care they are receiving continue to get the same bad care. Those who do complain might see an improvement.

There's no question that if it were not for the protection offered by unions, the workers in the hospital would be taken advantage of. Just ask the medical residents in training. However, it seems to me that it has become too hard to fire or even to discipline people who are simply not doing their jobs. There are too many folks talking on the phone for half the working day, too many who blast their music on the floors of the wards, who do crossword puzzles all day and sleep through the night shift. These people bring down the morale of the entire staff. Some sort of disciplinary administrative panel consisting of doctors, administrators, and a union rep is needed, one that can meet on a moment's notice and get rid of workers who are not doing their job. Otherwise, the phones will continue to ring for minute after minute, and the patients will not be fed or cleaned or taken to the bathroom. This is crucial. As a sign of our common humanity, we must strive to correct this blight on hospitals all across this country. Most of us will end up in the hospital one day, so if we don't act now, when we need some decent care we won't be able to get it.

As a youth, I often dreamed of being a comedian, and at times it is humor and sarcasm that enable me to cope with the horrors of working in hospitals. When the phones are ringing off the hook and the clerks are not picking them up, I've gone to the microphone, and over the loudspeaker I've requested that if there is anyone who is being paid to work here and would be willing to answer some of the phones, please do so at this time. But there are times when I can only shake my head in despair, as when I was told in no uncertain terms by the admitting clerk in a local emergency room to stop examining the patient so they could finish getting his insurance information. How can you answer a request like that? Believe me, the meek among us physicians actually walk away and wait. I told this clown to leave and come back later.

About three years ago, I upset every administrator and many of the physicians at my hospital when I refused to allow the doctors to transfer a patient named Ann from the intensive care unit to the medical floor. It seemed to me that the hospital and some of its staff had decided that she had outlived her welcome in the

ICU. She'd been there a month, and it was time to send her to the floor, where she had a good chance of dying. Silly me. I scared the staff into doing what was right for the patient. I wrote notes in the chart to document what I meant and put names in it as well, since as I explained earlier the chart is in fact a legal document. I even told those in charge I would call the district attorney's office if they sent her off the ICU (not that I knew how to get in touch with them). Ann stayed in the ICU and got the care she deserved. Rather than go to a floor to die, she left the hospital about a month later and went back to her life in Westchester, New York. I made a few enemies, got a few pats on the back, and got the great feeling that I had made a difference. But my guess is that most of my colleagues would have been too afraid or too uncaring to do what I did. And that may be why no one else has written a book like this before now.

I told you not to be taken in by ads and to distrust most of the things you see in the media. Hospitals try to sell themselves. Their idealized self-portrait is often in direct contradiction to real life. For me, it all comes down to finding a doctor you can trust, someone who has the decency to tell you where to go for your care, even if it isn't at the hospital where he or she admits patients. Primary-care doctors who work exclusively for a hospital and only send you to other physicians who work exclusively for that same hospital should be avoided. As I have mentioned, many of them are harangued and intimidated by their superiors with the message never to send patients out of the system.

Once in a hospital, don't assume that you can't leave. If you are unhappy with the care, the cleanliness, or the physicians who are caring for you, consider going to another hospital. Remember that you might need to pay for an ambulance to take you elsewhere, but consider it money well spent if your life is at stake.

And make sure you really need to be admitted in the first place. I hope that after this book is published, doctors will admit publicly for the first time that they are pressured to admit patients. Again, admitting patients reduces the hospital's exposure to responsibility (in the event that an error in judgment is made and a patient gets sick after leaving) and also fills what might have otherwise been empty beds. In the end, however, this hurts everyone. First, your premiums soar because of the unnecessary expense incurred by admitting all these extra patients. Second, by filling the beds with patients that don't need to be there, emergency rooms get crowded with patients. When a hospital has no empty beds you might be forced to spend an entire day on a stretcher in a noisy, impersonal ER in addition to being sick with perhaps a stroke, pneumonia, or who knows what ailment, life-threatening or not.

The solution to this problem is quite difficult. An insurance company cannot deny admissions if a doctor deems it necessary, but it can reward those hospitals, based on comparisons with similar hospitals in the area, that admit fewer patients with similar relatively benign forms of illness. Caps on malpractice rewards might also reduce the number of unnecessary admissions, since one of the primary motivations for admitting so many patients is the old "if we miss something, we'll get sued for millions" excuse.

Even if you are happy with your care, tell all the researchers who approach you to get lost. Avoid the temptation of enrolling in any drug or device study unless you and your doctor feel there are no other alternatives. I've told you that doctors who conduct research are paid anywhere from $2,000 to $5,000 for each patient they sign up. You on the other hand are getting nothing except the risk. Unless you have an illness that cannot be treated and you still wish to take a one-in-a-million chance at being an experiment, I would never even allow researchers to bother you.

Make sure your attending and not just one of his or her students comes to see you every day. And never be afraid to ask questions about your care and to expect appropriate answers. I understand that even in many of the elite hospitals, perhaps because of the huge patient load, much of the patient care is now delegated to the hospital residents. I've been told that the attendings don't visit the patients on weekends. So if you do go to a special cancer or heart hospital or use the top-notch doctor in your area, make sure before you are admitted for treatment that your doctor will come and see you every day. For the most part there is no magic in medicine, just hands-on care and trying to do the best for the patient. No matter how brilliant your doctor might be, he or she cannot take care of you from home or via cellular phone. This same advice also goes to all of you who have a regular physician. If he or the hospital he works for has decided to delegate his responsibility to other doctors, such as hospitalists, I'd think about choosing another doctor.

When a patient leaves the hospital his physician is required to write or dictate a discharge summary. I'd request a copy of that document before you leave. I would also make sure the nurse reviews all the medications you are expected to take when you get home, and if your doctor is really nice, I would ask him to call in your prescriptions to the pharmacy. The last thing you wish to do after being discharged from the hospital is wait for an hour while the pharmacist fills your prescription. And if you are going to a rehab center or nursing home, I'd make sure someone in the family has checked it out first. Finally, I'd leave the hospital when you're ready to leave, not when some nursing supervisor or administrator tells you and your doctor you should leave.

As far as outpatient care goes, it's important to take your time when choosing your doctor. I'd scrutinize the tips I gave you earlier, including simple things that you can do from home. If you are pleased with your research, I'd consider your first appointment a trial. If the doctor seems to be honest, if he and his staff are courteous, and the office is clean and well run, then I guess you've got a new doctor. But on the other hand, if the doctor has too many gimmicks up his sleeve, suggests all sorts of tests on the first trial visit, and does all his labs in his office (like blood work and unethical sonograms), well, that is an even easier decision: Leave and never go back. And by the way, if your doctor does send your blood to a lab, make sure it's a well-respected lab. Have them send a copy of your results straight to you. I've heard of several cases where, in a busy office, a doctor misdiagnosed an abnormal lab report.

I'd avoid all physicians and imaging centers that advertise on TV. And those imaging centers that tell you they can find microscopic cancers and heart disease more often find nothing, or worse, may scare you half to death with some erroneous finding.

I remain somewhat conflicted and even apprehensive about how I have portrayed some of my colleagues and the institutions where they work. For it is also certainly the case that some of the brightest, most dedicated, and most honest people in our country are physicians. These gifted men and women should be treated as a precious part of our society, but today it seems that many are not. They must contend with the insurance companies, the malpractice payments, the arrogant chiefs of the hospital and their sycophants, and the malpractice lawyers. It's a very tough environment to work in, and I'm afraid many of us are coping with our responsibilities instead of enjoying them.

Some doctors have seen their fees cut by more than half over the past ten years. Add inflation and the expense of maintaining a practice and paying malpractice premiums, and you've got a huge reduction in salary.

If the medical environment I have described remains the same, I believe fewer and fewer of America's gifted youths will go into the study of medicine, and the ones who do study medicine will choose the most lucrative specialties, very often the fee-for-service jobs like dermatology and plastic surgery. An excellent example of this trend involves the field of cardiothoracic surgery. It would be my hope that only the most intelligent and gifted physicians would go into this field, but instead, a recent statement by the *Society of Thoracic Surgeons* notes "that at the beginning of 2003 the National Residency Matching Program has reported that 21 out of 144 positions offered in cardiothoracic surgery have not been filled."[3] In other words, they can't even find enough residents from American and/or foreign schools who even wish to be CT surgeons. Not surprisingly, it is the specialties with cushier lifestyles and huge fee-for-service salaries that have become the most competitive.

We need to encourage our best students to go into medicine, and once in the field, to choose the areas of specialization that our society needs.

First, I would put limits on the amount medical schools can charge for tuition. You may not be aware of this, but it's only in the first two years that students are actually in classrooms. For the next two years most medical students are working in hospitals, assisting the doctors (and sometimes even acting as doctors), even while they must continue to pay their tuition, which can run well over $30,000 per year.

Second, our society needs to put some kind of cap on the torrent of "pain-and-suffering" malpractice awards and redefine what we consider malpractice to be in the first place. Fines should be levied to penalize lawyers who attempt to bring frivolous, cynical, but no less damaging suits to court. There should also be an easy mechanism in place that enables doctors to sue them in return. Tasteless advertisements by lawyers should be stopped. And to those powerful groups of lawyers and their political friends, I say, *Have you no decency?* How can our society, enlightened in so many ways, not stop the constantly escalating increases in malpractice insurance when we know we are going to drive our doctors right out of their practices and out of medicine altogether? In the state of California, it has been proven that if you limit payments for pain and suffering in medical malpractice cases and, equally important, put some kind of price controls on the malpractice insurance carriers (so the insurance companies don't just make more and more money), you can substantially diminish the cost of medical malpractice insurance.

Yet in arguments by these same plaintiffs' lawyers (many of whom don't accept cases where they don't see a million-dollar-plus settlement), they suggest we might just put caps on what the doctors have to pay, since if you look at the premiums doctors paid in California, they really didn't drop till that final legislation act was enacted. How cynical can these folks be? Obviously if we continue to allow multimillion-dollar malpractice payments and also put price controls on what malpractice insurers can charge, something must give way. Surely it will be that all the malpractice insurers in our country will cease doing business, since they'll all lose money. While this isn't a perfect solution—some people won't be able to find a malpractice attorney who will take a case for a paltry potential award of $250,000— we do need to make these changes soon.

Third, the Justice Department together with some sort of organization of self-policing physicians should hunt down the criminal elements of the profession and make them pay back every penny of their ill-gotten gains.

Fourth, related to the above, doctors should no longer be able or be permitted to perform any studies, farm out those studies, or bill for any procedures of any kind other than what they were trained and certified to do. In other words, if you are not board certified in a given discipline, you should not be able to practice that type of medicine. A general practitioner or an internist, in other words, should not be performing colonoscopies, stress tests, or any type of sonography. A special code can be given to those doctors who meet the requirements, like board certification, and should be mandatory when they bill for any of these special studies or consultations. In sparsely populated areas of our country, where the nearest specialist might be hours away, technicians could be trained to perform the examinations, and those studies read via modem set up by properly trained physicians. In my opinion it is just as dangerous to allow a doctor who is not trained to interpret a test as to have no test done at all. And as I mentioned, these costly tests and examinations and machines are costing our insurers and thus ourselves (through skyrocketing premiums) billions of dollars a year.

Fifth, physicians who specialize in fee-for-service cosmetic procedures should be forced to pay a luxury tax, which I suggest should be a percentage of their fee. The money saved through these penalties and taxes could go back into the health-care system to maintain reasonable pay for doctors and provide some health insurance for the working poor.

Finally, I want to go on the record saying that not all of the reductions in doctor reimbursement are wrong. Many Medicare fees for procedures have fallen substantially over the years, but at the same time, some of these procedures are performed more and more frequently and with greater and greater ease thanks to advances in technology. For example, Medicare paid twice as much for a cataract operation in the 1980s as it does today (around $800 per eye), but the surgery is now very simple for a quality surgeon and many of these surgeons can perform ten, or even twenty, procedures in one day. At $800 per surgery, that's as much as $16,000 for one day's work. The recent increase in indications for colonoscopy have also increased the frequency with which this test is performed, but again, in my opinion, the reduction in charge has not been totally unfair.

We need to set up reasonable standards for malpractice, and the doctors who fall outside these limits should be punished. Their licenses to practice should be suspended, or they should be given a period of probation at the very least. And for those who perform illegal and unethical procedures, there should be huge fines (which go to the citizens and not the lawyers). Incarceration should even be considered in the most egregious and harmful cases. However, we should not penalize a doctor who had one death out of a thousand during a surgical procedure when the average death rate for the identical procedure is 1 percent.

I hope that you have learned a lot about this secretive and cloistered profession. I've tried to give you the inside story, to tell you about the sick condition of the medical profession as truthfully as I can, but, most important, to give you tools to help you get the best possible medical care. For those who will condemn this book, most likely the duplicitous types I have written about, I can only say that I understand your position. Perhaps this will be the beginning of the end of the greatest rip-off ever imposed on the American consumer.

Notes

Introduction

1. *http://www.thoracicrad.org.* Society of Thoracic Radiology.

2. Moseley JB, O'Malley K, Peterson NJ, et al. "A Controlled Trial of Arthroscopic Surgery for Osteoarthritis of the Knee." *New England Journal of Medicine* 2002; 347:81–88.

3. Personal communication with New-York Presbyterian Hospital.

4. "Two Brothers Confront Columbia over Payment of a 'Dean's Tax.'" *New York Times,* December 23, 2002.

Chapter 1. How to Choose Your Doctor

1. *Who in Medicine and Healthcare,* 2002–2004, 4th ed., Marquis Publishing.

2. Edelman, S. "Hospital Heartache," *New York Post,* December 15, 2002.

3. Ibid.

4. *http://www.phc4.org/idb/Cabg/default.cfm.* Pennsylvania Health Care Cost Containment Council. Pennsylvania's Guide to Coronary Artery Bypass Graft (CABG) Surgery, 2000.

5. Ibid.

6. *http://www.health.state.ny.us/home.html*. New York State Department of Health.

7. "CASS principal investigators and their associates: Myocardial infarction and mortality in the Coronary Artery Surgery Study (CASS) randomized trial," *New England Journal of Medicine* 1984; 310:750–758.

8. "The Veterans Administration coronary artery bypass surgery cooperative study group: Eleven-year survival in the Veterans Administration randomized trial of coronary bypass surgery for stable angina," *New England Journal of Medicine* 1984; 311:1333–1339.

9. Varnauskas E. "Survival, myocardial infarction, and employment status in a prospective randomized study of coronary bypass surgery," *Circulation* 1985; 72(Suppl 5): 90.

10. Yasuf S, Zucker D, Peduzzi P, et al. "Effect of coronary artery bypass surgery on survival; Overview of 10-year results from randomized trials by the Coronary Artery Bypass Surgery Trialists Collaboration," *Lancet* 1994; 344:563.

11. Eagle KA, Guyton RA, et al. "ACC/AHA Guidelines for coronary artery bypass graft surgery. A report of the American College of Cardiology/American Heart Association task force on practice guidelines," *Journal of the American College of Cardiology* 1999; 34(4): 1262–1347.

12. Peterson, ED, DeLong ER, Jollis JG, et al. "The effects of New York's bypass surgery provider profiling on access to care and patient outcomes in the elderly," *Journal of the American College of Cardiology* 1998; 32(4): 993–999.

Chapter 2. How to Survive Your Hospital Stay

1. Personal source and interview with JCAHO.

2. Ibid.

3. Interview with hospital administrator.

4. Department of Medicine, Montefiore Hospital. "AOS service memo."

5. Centers for Disease Control and Prevention. "Guidelines for the prevention of intravascular catheter-related infections," *Morbidity and Monthly Weekly Report* 2002:51 (No.RR-10): 1–21.

6. Ibid.

7. Maki DG. "Engineering out the risk of infection with urinary catheters," *Emerging Infectious Diseases* 2001; 7(2): 1–6.

8. Ibid.

9. Pollack C, Tapson V, Birnbaumer D, et al. "The clinical challenge of venous thromboembolism (VTE) in the hospitalized patient: Optimizing recognition, evaluation, and prophylasix of at-risk patients. Centers of Excellence," *Venous and Arterial Thrombosis Panel Reports.* November 1, 2002:1–13.

10. Kilcullen JK, Deshpande KS, Kvetan V. Chapter 216: "Transport of the critically ill patient." In Irwin and Rippe (eds). *Intensive Care Medicine,* 5th ed. 2003: 2258–2266.

11. Personal source and interview with hospital administrator.

Chapter 3. Tricks of the Trade—How Some Doctors
Are Taking Advantage of You and the System

1. At the time this memo was written these doctors worked for the hospital. I am not criticizing the qualifications of these surgeons. In fact Dr. Richard Brodman became one of the most gifted surgeons I've encountered and even saved my grandfather's life several years ago. He is now chief of cardiothoracic surgery at the University of Buffalo.

2. Bashore TM, Bates ER, Berger PB, et al. American College of Cardiology/ Society for Cardiac Angiography and Interventions. "Clinical expert consensus document on catheterization laboratory standards," *Journal of American College of Cardiology* 2001; 37(8): 2170–2214.

3. Scanlon PI, Faxon DP. "ACC/AHA Guidelines for coronary angiography," *Journal of American College of Cardiology* 1999; 33(6): 1756–1824.

4. Smith SC, Dove JT, Jacobs AK, et al. ACC/AHA "Guidelines for percutaneous coronary intervention," *Circulation* 2001; 103:3019–3041.

5. Op. cit.

6. Imperiale TF, Wagner DG, Lin CY, et al. "Risk of advanced proximal neoplasms in asymptomatic adults according to the distal colorectal findings," *New England Journal of Medicine* 2000; 343: 169–174.

7. Liberman DA, Weiss DG, Bond JH, et al. "Use of colonoscopy to screen asymptomatic adults for colorectal cancer," *New England Journal of Medicine* 2000; 343: 162–168.

8. Schlant RC, Adolph RJ, DiMarco JP, et al. "Guidelines for electrocardiography. A report of the American College of Cardiology/American Heart Association Task Force on Assessment of Diagnostic and Therapeutic Cardiovascular Procedures," *Journal of the American College of Cardiology* 1992; 19: 473–481.

9. Gibbons RJ, Balady GJ, Beasley JW, et al. "ACC/AHA Guidelines for exercise testing. A report of the American College of Cardiology/American Heart Association Task Force on Practice Guidelines," *Journal of the American College of Cardiology* 1997; 30: 260–315.

10. Schwartz JA, Lui G, and Brooks SC. "Genistein-mediated attenuation of tamoxifen induced antagonism from estrogen receptor regulated genes," *Biochem. Biophys. Res. Comm.* 1998; 253:38–43.

11. Gianelli DM. "Ethics council revisits office-based product sales," *American Medical Association News*, June 7, 1999; 1–5.

12. Ibid.

Notes

Chapter 5. Should I Take Part in a Scientific Study?

1. Morin K, Rakatansky H, Riddick FA, et al. "Managing conflicts of interest in the conduct of clinical trials, *Journal of the American Medical Association* 2002; 287: 78–84.

2. Lind S. "Financial issues and incentives related to clinical research and innovative therapies," in Vanderpool HY. *The Ethics of Research Involving Human Subjects: Facing the 21st Century.* (Hagerstown, MD: University Publishing Group; 1996), 185–202.

3. Foy R, Parry J, McAvoy B. "Clinical trials in primary care. Targeting payments for trials might help improve recruitment and quality," *British Medical Journal* 1998; 317:185–202.

4. Cauchon D. "FDA Advisers tied to industry," *USA Today.* September 25, 2000, p 01A.

5. Willman D. "Posicor: 143 deaths did not stop approval," *Los Angeles Times.* December 20, 2000.

6. "The TIMI-3B investigators. Thrombolysis in Myocardial Ischemia-3B," *Circulation* 1994: 89: 1545–1556.

7. Van de Werf F, Baim DS. "Reperfusion for ST-segment elevation myocardial infarction. An overview of current treatment options," *Circulation* 2002; 105: 2813–2816.

8. Weaver WD, Simes RJ, Betriu A, et al. "Comparison of primary coronary angioplasty and intravenous thrombolytics therapy of acute myocardial infarction: A quantitative review," *Journal of the American Medical Association* 1997; 278: 2093–2098.

9. *http://www.timi.org.* TIMI Study Group.

10. Anderson HR. "Danish trial in acute myocardial infarction (DANAMI-2)." Presented at *American College of Cardiology Scientific Sessions.* Atlanta, GA; March 20, 2002.

11. Anderson HR, Nielsen TT, Rasmussen K, et al. "A comparison of coronary angioplasty with fibrinolytic therapy in acute myocardial infarction, *New England Journal of Medicine* 2003; 349: 733–742.

12. Widimsky P. "The PRAGUE results." Presented at the European Society of Cardiology. Berlin, Germany; September 1, 2002.

13. Ibid.

14. Grines CL, Westerhausen DR, Grines LL, et al., for the Air PAMI Study Group, "A randomized trial of transfer for primary angioplasty versus on-site thrombolysis in patients with high-risk myocardial infarction. The air primary angioplasty in myocardial infarction study," *Journal of the American College of Cardiology* 2002; 39: 1713–1719.

15. Ibid.

16. Antman EM, Braunwald E. Chapter 35: "Acute Myocardial Infarction." In Braunwald E, Zipes DP, Libby P (eds). *Heart Disease*, 6th ed. Philadelphia, PA: W.B. Saunders; 2001: 1153.

17. "The cardia arrhythmia suppression trial (CAST) Investigators. Preliminary report: Effect of encainide and flecainide on mortality in a randomized trial of arrhythmia suppression after myocardial infarction," *New England Journal of Medicine* 1989; 321:406–412.

18. Ibid.

19. Waldo AL, Camm AJ, deRuyter H, et al. "The SWORD trial. Effect of d-sotalol on mortality in patients with left ventricular dysfunction after recent and remote myocardial infarction," *Lancet* 1996; 348:7–12.

20. Ibid.

21. The CONSENSUS Trial Study Group. "Effects of enalapril on mortality in severe congestive heart failure. Results of the Cooperative North Scandinavian Enalapril Survival Study (CONSENSUS)." *New England Journal of Medicine* 1987; 316:1429–1435.

22. Brenner BM, Cooper ME, de Zeeuw D, et al. The RENAAL Study Investi-

gators. "Effects of Losartan on renal and cardiovascular outcomes in patients with type 2 diabetes and nephropathy," *New England Journal of Medicine* 2001; 345: 861–869.

23. Dagenais GR, Yusuf S, Bourassa MG, et al. "Effects of Ramipril on the coronary events in high-risk persons: Results of the Heart Outcomes Prevention Evaluation (HOPE) Study," *Circulation* 2001; 104: 522–526.

24. Ibid.

25. Lewis EJ, Hunsicker LG, Bain BP, et al, for the Collaborative Study Group. "The effect of angiotensin-converting-enzyme inhibition of diabetic nephropathy," *New England Journal of Medicine* 1993; 329:1456–1462.

26. The RENAAL Study Investigators.

27. The HOPE Investigators.

28. Bristow MR, Port JD, Kelly RA. Chapter 18. "Treatment of heart failure: Pharmacologic methods," in Braunwald E, Zipes DP, Libby P (eds). *Heart Disease*, 6th ed. Philadelphia, PA: W.B. Saunders; 2001: 562–599.

29. Peterson P, Boysen G, Godtfredsen J, et al. The Copenhagen AFASAK Study. "Placebo-controlled, randomized trial of warfarin and aspirin for prevention of thromboembolic complication in chronic atrial fibrillation," *Lancet* 1989; 1: 175–179.

30. SPAF Investigators. "Preliminary report of the Stroke Prevention in Atrial Fibrillation study," *New England Journal of Medicine* 1990; 322: 863–868.

31. "The Boston Area Anticoagulation Trial for Atrial Fibrillation investigators (BAATAF) investigators: The effect of low-dose warfarin on the risk of stroke in patients with nonrheumatic atrial fibrillation," *New England Journal of Medicine* 1990; 323: 1505–1511.

32. Connolly SJ, Laupacis A, Gent M, et al. "Canadian Atrial Fibrillation Anticoagulation (CAFA) study," *Journal of the American Journal of Cardiology* 1991; 18: 349–355.

33. Ezekowitz MD, Bridges SL, James KE, et al. "Warfarin in the prevention of stroke associated with nonrheumatic atrial fibrillation. Veterans Affairs stroke prevention in nonrheumatic atrial fibrillation (SPINAF) Investigators," *New England Journal of Medicine* 1992; 327: 1406–1412.

34. "The European Atrial Fibrillation Trial (EAFT) investigators. Secondary prevention in nonrheumatic atrial fibrillation after transient ischemic attack or minor stroke," *Lancet* 1993; 342: 1255–1262.

Chapter 6. The Pharmaceutical Industry

1. *http://info@familiesusa.org*. Families USA, NW Washington DC.

2. *http://www.imshealth.org*. IMS, Fairfield, CT.

3. *http://www.merck.com*. Merck & Co., Inc., Whitehouse Station, NJ.

4. Associated Press. "US psychiatrists concern over drug sales reps sitting in on treatments," January 20, 2003.

5. Ibid.

6. *http://oig.hhs.gov*. Office of Inspector Control. Voluntary Compliance Guidance Issued for Pharmaceutical Manufacturers. April 28, 2003.

7. Ibid.

8. 2003 Pfizer Annual Report.

9. The ALLHAT Officers and Coordinators for the ALLHAT Collaborative Research Group. "Major outcomes in high-risk hypertensive patients randomized to angiotensin-converting enzyme inhibitor or calcium channel blocker vs diuretic: The Antihypertensive and Lipid-Lowering treatment to prevent Heart Attack Trial (ALLHAT)," *Journal of the American Medical Association* 2002; 288: 2981–2997.

10. Ibid.

11. Grodstein F, Stampfer MJ, Colditz, GA, et al. "Post menopausal hormone therapy and mortality," *New England Journal of Medicine* 1997; 336: 1769–1775.

12. Susan M. Love, Karen Lindsey (Contributor). *Dr. Susan Love's Hormone Book: Making Informed Choices About Menopause* (Three Rivers Press, 1997).

13. Ibid.

14. Gladwell M. "The estrogen question: How wrong is Dr. Susan Love?" *The New Yorker,* June 9, 1997.

15. Hulley S, Grady D, Bush T, et al. "Heart and Estrogen/Progestin Replacement Study (HERS) research group. Randomized trial of estrogen plus progestin for secondary prevention of coronary disease in postmenopausal women," *Journal of the American Medical Association* 1998; 280: 605–613.

16. Writing Group for the Women's Health Initiative (WHI) Investigators. "Risks and benefits of estrogen plus progestin in healthy postmenopausal women: Results from the Women's Health Initiative randomized controlled trial," *Journal of the American Medical Association* 2002; 288: 321–333.

17. Saftlas H. "Wyeth: Ready to rebound," Insight from Standard & Poor's *Business Week Online,* September 16, 2002.

18. Stephenson J. "FDA orders estrogen safety warnings: Agency offers guidance for HRT use," *Journal of the American Medical Association* 2004; 289 (5): 537–538.

19. Press Release. Wyeth Pharmaceuticals, Madison, NJ: June 9, 2003.

20. Product Information: Zocor, simvastatin. Merck & Co. Inc., Whitehouse Station, NJ: April 2003.

21. *Red Book: Drug Topics.* Thompson Micromedex. (Montvale, NJ: April 2003).

22. Cohen M, Demers C, Gurfinkel EP, et al. "Efficacy and safety of subcutaneous enoxaparin in non-q-wave coronary events," *New England Journal of Medicine* 1997; 337: 447–452.

23. Klein W, Buchwald A, Hillis SE. "Comparison of low-molecular-weight heparin with unfractioned heparin acutely and with placebo for 6 weeks in

the management of unstable coronary artery disease: Fragmin In unstable Coronary artery disease study (FRIC)," *Circulation* 1997; 96: 61–68.

24. *http://drugstore.com*

25. *http://www.coumadinsettlement.com.* Warfarin Sodium Antitrust Consumer and Third Party Payor Settlement. November 4, 2002.

26. Op. cit.

27. *http://canada-pharmacy.com*

28. Moore, TJ. *Deadly Medicine: Why Tens of Thousands of Heart Patients Died in America's Worst Drug Disaster* (Simon & Schuster, March 1995).

29. Cauchon, D. "FDA advisers tied to industry." *USA Today,* Oct. 1, 2000.

30. Cohn JN, Archibald DG, Ziesche S, et al. "Effect of vasodilator therapy on mortality in chronic congestive heart failure," *New England Journal of Medicine* 1986; 314: 1547–1552.

31. Poole-Wilson PA, Swedberg K, Cleland JGF, et al, for the COMET Investigators. "Comparison of carvedilol and metoprolol on clinical outcomes in patients with chronic heart failure in the Carvedilol or Metoprolol European Trial (COMET): a randomized controlled trial," *Lancet.* 2003; 362: 7–13.

32. Magill-Lewis J. "New Pill Splitting Study Yields Surprising Results," *Drug Topics.* February 18, 2002: 20.

33. Stafford RS, Radley DC. "The potential of pill splitting to achieve cost savings," *The American Journal of Managed Care* 2002; 8 (8): 706–712.

34. Pfizer Annual Financial Report 2002.

35. *http://dcc2.bumc.bu.edu/hs/ushealthreform.html.* Sager A, Socolar D. "Americans would save $38 billion in 2001 if we paid Canadian prices for brand name prescription drugs." Revised written version of testimony before the Subcommittee on Consumer Affairs, Foreign Commerce, and Tourism, Committee on Commerce, Science, and Transportation U.S. Senate. September 5, 2001.

36. Pitt B, Zannad F, Remme WJ, et al. "The Randomized Aldactone Evaluation Study Investigators (RALES): The effect of spironolactone on morbidity and mortality in patients with severe heart failure," *New England
Journal of Medicine 1999*; 341: 709–17.

37. National Institute for Health Care Management. "Prescription drugs and
mass media advertising," Sept. 2000: 1–8.

38. *http://www.imshealth.org.* IMS, Fairfield, CT.

Chapter 7. Medicine in Crisis

1. *http://www.acponline.org/college/pressroom/michiganhmo.htm.* American
College of Physicians. Press Release: Michigan HMO Sets Limits on Patient Choices of Primary Care Physicians. January 4, 2001.

2. *http://www.medicarerights.org.* Hayes, RM. Press Release from the Medicare Rights Center, January 28, 2003.

Conclusion

1. *http://dcc2.bumc.bu.edu/hs/ushealthreform.html.* Sager A, Socolar D.
"Americans would save $38 billion in 2001 if we paid Canadian prices for
brand name prescription drugs." Revised written version of testimony be-
fore the Subcommittee on Consumer Affairs, Foreign Commerce, and
Tourism, Committee on Commerce, Science, and Transportation U.S. Senate.
September 5, 2001.

2. Stolberg SG. "House passes drug bill; battle is likely in Senate," *New York
Times* July 26, 2003: Section A, Pg 11.

3. *http://www.sts.org.* The Society of Thoracic Surgeons. "Shortage of new
heart surgeons predicted," August 6, 2002.

Acknowledgments

I have been privileged to know some very special people who have taught me life's lessons in the most important way: They didn't even know they had done so. My grandma, Lillian Marks, was one such person. She passed away during my first years of college, from a cancer that her gynecologist missed and that was possibly caused by the estrogen replacement therapy she had received "to make her feel better." She taught me how special grandmas are. At the end of a hard day it is not always easy for many of us to treat some of our sick and elderly patients with compassion, but I am always reminded of the kindness Grandma possessed and how I always treated her with the respect and honor she deserved. I take the memory of her with me wherever I go, and she helps me to be compassionate. I miss her vegetable soup, her calling out to my grandpa, Murray, to come into the house, and I thank her for always lifting me up when I thought I was not good enough, strong enough, or smart enough to do something worthwhile. I guess that's what grandmas do for you. I only wish that I had been far enough along in my career to have helped her—as I did Grandpa Murray—live into her nineties.

I met Mie Hyashi during my training in cardiology at Montefiore. She was a bright-eyed Japanese-American woman, immensely intelligent but also kind and humble. We became great friends and even traveled a bit together. Mie taught me how nice it is to do simple things in life, to be content, and to find happiness in my job. She left New York a few years ago, fell back in love with a college sweetheart, and had a baby boy. But Mie was too kind and beautiful for this world, and she passed on less than a year after becoming a mother. I had lost touch with her, but I felt her presence at her memorial, which was held in New York this past winter. I only hope that I can someday be as caring and humble as Mie was.

There are so many others who give me the impetus to be my best. First, of course, my mom and dad, who worked so hard to keep me happy and healthy as a child. My precious Amanda, who brings pure joy and love into our home, and "our children," Toby and Shmoby, who through their soft purrs and warm cuddles in the middle of a cold New York night help me forget the terrible things I see and write about in this book. My friends and partners in my practice, Stu, Meir, and Richard, with whom I often consult about patients and about life. And those great nurses, nurse practitioners, and physician assistants I work with who bring the same caring and energy to work every day, even though many of them work in an almost intolerable system. And finally, some of the kindest people I have ever met: the physicians who trust me to take care of their patients but ask nothing in return—there are too many to mention here.

Allen Peacock came to see me as a patient, but after hearing my idea and reading a cursory outline, he became my editor, coach, advocate, and friend. My agent, Ron Bard, a.k.a. the Psychic, who believed in me as a doctor and a writer, introduced me to his Northeast Media Group and to David Highfill and Marilyn Ducksworth, the fine people at G. P. Putnam's Sons—where this all became possible.